PRACTICAL DIABETES

Second edition

David Levy MD FRCP
Consultant Physician
Gillian Hanson Centre
Whipps Cross University Hospital
London

ALTMAN

Published by Altman Publishing, 7 Ash Copse, Bricket Wood, St Albans, Herts, AL2 3YA, UK

First edition 1999, published by Greenwich Medical Media Ltd, London
Second edition 2006

Typeset in 10/12 Optima by Scribe Design Ltd, Ashford, Kent
Printed in Great Britain by Ingersoll Printers Ltd, Wembley

ISBN 1 86036 033 5

A catalogue record for this book is available from the British Library

∞ Printed on acid-free text paper, manufactured in accordance with ANSI/NISO Z39.48-1992 (Permanence of Paper)

CONTENTS

Colour plates appear between pp. 114 and 115

PREFACE

The modest success of the first edition of *Practical Diabetes* (1999) now seems distant, but the intervening 6 years have not generated the revolutions in practical aspects of diabetes management that we imagined in our generally overheated pre-millennial state. The march of the reports of the mega-drug trials, mostly started, in their dozens, in the mid- and late-1990s, has continued, sometimes with perverse, or at least non-consistent, outcomes, fuelling uncertainty for practitioners and the guideline industry alike. The latter has, no surprise here, grown to the point at which 50+-page reports thud (at least with the electronic equivalent of a thud) several times a week onto my computer desktop. The confident assertion in late 1998 that ALLHAT, the most mega of all the mega-hypertension trials, would prove definitive, didn't turn out to be anything of the kind, and became mired in controversy even before its final publication in 2002. Likewise, the flurry of trials designed to support the concept of 'added benefit' of particular agents or groups of agents has supported the view that statins work through LDL lowering, and antihypertensive agents work through, well, BP lowering. ASCOT-BPLA (2005) will probably change our prescribing habits, though getting BP to lower targets is still more important than the agents used. However, the most recent statin studies have moved high-sensitivity CRP into the realm of a risk factor independent of LDL, although again hinting very strongly that no LDL level is too low for our highest risk patients. The heroic DIGAMI 2 study, another study that would finally determine practice once and for all, this time in relation to glycaemic control in diabetic heart attack patients, reported in September 2004, and its shadowy conclusions sadly encapsulated many of the difficulties of independent clinical trial work in the modern era, uncovering more questions than answers, but fundamentally reinforcing the view that coronary outcomes in type 2 diabetes can be dramatically improved – through persistent, rather non-dramatic, but systematic interventions, including vigorous percutaneous and coronary bypass procedures. Of course, targets have continued to fall, especially lipids, though those for glycaemic control, as frustratingly difficult to deal with as they were in 1999, remain merely a huge challenge. That challenge, at least in type 1 diabetes, has been met in small part with the advent of insulin analogues, most impressively with the long-acting analogues, and useful techniques like continuous glucose monitoring studies. Sadly, continuous subcutaneous insulin infusion (CSII) treatment, standard therapy in much of the rest of the Western world, remains very patchily available in the UK, and we remain in the foothills (or perhaps the offshore islands) of pancreatic and islet-cell transplantation.

The most interesting trials, published in a concise cohort over the past 6 years, and conceived in the early 1990s, have investigated prevention (or delay) of type 2 diabetes by studying patients with impaired glucose tolerance. Their simple message, that intensive lifestyle intervention is the most effective tool, will not translate into a slowing of the type 2 diabetes epidemic until we finally begin to understand the appalling consequences of this condition when untreated. For a shocking account of the devastating effects of acculturation leading to epidemic diabetes in a high-risk population, read the tragic tale of the Micronesian island of Naurua in *Fat Wars* by Ellen Ruppel Shell (Penguin, 2004). I have included a table of clinical trials reporting up to 2005, though I have not described most of them in detail as in the first edition. Medline (www.nlm.nih.gov) is a much more informative source; the trial acronym plus 'diabetes' is likely to lead you to the detailed reference for the main studies. I have, however, quoted a few websites that might be of interest.

Concepts have moved on rapidly, their uptake less so. The idea of insulin resistance and the associated metabolic syndrome, central to both type 1 and type 2 diabetes, and now old (1988) has been defined and defined again. The most recent proposal (IDF, 2005), likely to be endorsed worldwide, raises substantial practical questions about the possible impact of more glucose tolerance tests by reducing the criterion for normal fasting glucose to 5.5 mmol/L or lower, but I may have pre-empted the experts here, and I hope I have not caused more confusion than there already is. Regardless, practitioners seem not to be able to easily translate the concept of insulin resistance into therapeutic benefit for patients, despite the overwhelming evidence of its importance, and the advent of safe thiazolidinediones (glitazones). Understanding insulin resistance/metabolic syndrome clarifies much that has previously been mysterious in diabetes; it has drawn non-alcoholic fatty liver disease, the polycystic ovarian syndrome, non-diabetic coronary heart disease, obstructive sleep apnoea, gout and other important diseases into the metabolic sphere; and it also warns us about the serious consequences of acquired insulin resistance in our type 1 patients. The metabolic syndrome is so protean and widespread that I could not resist adding a short chapter, despite the cautionary backlash that appears to have started as I write this preface, re-articulating, among other matters, anxieties that have always been with us about whether a syndrome can be regarded as a disease. The practical implication of the metabolic syndrome – the need for intensive multifactorial intervention – found its expression in the wonderful Steno Type 2 study (2003), proof, if ever it were needed, that the single magic pill (even the polypill) will probably never be enough. The one concept that will certainly bloom therapeutically over the next few years is that of the enteric (gut) hormone system; the recognition of the incretin concept has led to the development of several important agents that will complement the treatments of insulin resistance and insulin deficiency in type 2 diabetes. Once this tranche of drugs is in place, we have nearly all the pharmacological tools we need to markedly delay or even prevent the devastating cardiovascular complications of type 2 diabetes. Translating these into a reduction, or even a stabilisation of end-stage diabetes complications in larger populations remains a huge challenge, because diet and exercise targets are much more difficult to achieve than near-undetectable LDL levels. One terminological whinge (indulge me): you won't find the word 'aggressive' in these pages. Barely a lecture or clinical trial report (or entry in the clinical notes of someone planning fluid replacement in a patient with diabetic ketoacidosis) emerges without someone trying to outdo their colleagues in the aggression with which they can treat their patients. I think I know what they are getting at, but diabetologists are not aggressive people, in general; neither are their patients, in general, and I think 'enthusiastic' or 'vigorous' conveys more what we are really trying to do without the risk of misunderstanding (and 'aggressive' fluid therapy in DKA/HHS often does serious harm).

This little volume again tries to bridge the divide between primary and secondary care diabetes by dealing with practical problems common to professionals who manage patients with diabetes. In particular, I hope I have been able to tackle some of the questions that hospital and general practice colleagues frequently ask me, and which are not usually addressed in the standard textbooks. As before, there are no hierarchical organisation diagrams, no Gant charts, no links to motivational websites, no statements of vision, mission or philosophy, no declarations of undying loyalty to the concept of quality (which goes without saying); others can do these kinds of things much better than me. But provision of diabetes care where it is best delivered is now rightly a question at the top of the agenda, and I am delighted that Dr Michal Grenville has contributed a chapter on the primary care approach to diabetes, in particular in relation to the National Service Framework for diabetes (2002) and the new GMS contract for General Practitioners. There is, of course, a risk that in trying to address all audiences, I will fail to satisfy any of them; not wishing to underplay the scale of this risk, I have introduced several chapters with an outline of basic mechanisms, just to remind us that pragmatism must always be tempered with a sound knowledge of basic physiology and pathology.

Victor Lawrence, a recent specialist registrar at Whipps Cross, got me re-thinking diabetic hyperglycaemic emergencies in a proper physiological way, and Chapter 3 owes much to his input. Laura Liew, senior Diabetes Specialist Nurse, helped with the shifting sands table of insulins, and acquired many digital photographs, a few of which are included. I remain very grateful to all the members of the clinical team, especially the podiatrists, at the Gillian Hanson Centre who have contributed so much clinical wisdom – some of which I hope you will find in these pages.

Peter Altman took up the challenge of publishing this second edition, and did so with continual good humour and patience, and occasional demonstrations of newly acquired skills as a member of the Magic Circle, rather splendidly having celebrated its centenary last year (unfortunately the magic doesn't extend to a text that writes itself). We agonised about changing the title to something with a little more pizzazz ('Diabetes at the Sharp End' was rejected, for reasons I still can't quite fathom, and sadly the glorious 'Diabetes for Dummies' had already been taken), but a key, if dour, British buzz-phrase of c.2001 – 'It does exactly what it says on the tin' – a reference to an advertisement for a proprietary wood varnish, not, fortunately, a whitewash – continually came to mind, and reinforced the retention of the previous name. If I have succeeded even in part in doing what it says on the tin, then I can cope with a mildly boring title.

David Levy
London, January 2006
David.Levy@Whippsx.nhs.uk

ABBREVIATIONS, STUDIES AND TRIALS

Abbreviations

A&E	Accident and Emergency
AACE	American Association of Clinical Endocrinologists
ABPM	ambulatory blood pressure measurement
ACE(i)	angiotensin converting enzyme (inhibitor)
ACR	albumin:creatinine ratio
ACS	acute coronary syndrome
ADA	American Diabetes Association
AER	albumin excretion rate
APS	autoimmune polyglandular syndrome
ARB	angiotensin receptor blocker ('sartans')
BMI	body mass index
BNF	British National Formulary
BP	blood pressure
CABG	coronary artery bypass graft
CAD	coronary artery disease
CAPD	continuous ambulatory peritoneal dialysis
CBG	capillary blood glucose
CCB	calcium channel blocker
CETP	cholesteryl ester transfer protein
CGMS	continuous glucose monitoring study
CHD	coronary heart disease
CK	creatine kinase
CRP	C-reactive protein
CSII	continuous subcutaneous insulin infusion (pump)
CSMO	clinically significant macular oedema
CVD	cardiovascular disease
DHA	docosahexanoic acid
DKA	diabetic ketoacidosis
DPP	dipeptidyl peptidase
ECG	electrocardiogram
EPA	eicosapentanoic acid
EPO	erythropoietin
ESR	erythrocyte sedimentation rate
ESRF	end-stage renal failure
FBC	full blood count
FPG	fasting (venous) plasma glucose
FSH	follicle-stimulating hormone

GAD	glutamic acid decarboxylase
GDM	gestational diabetes mellitus
GFR	glomerular filtration rate (eGFR estimated glomerular filtration rate)
GIK	glucose-insulin-potassium (infusion)
GIP	glucose-dependent insulinotropic polypeptide
GLA	gamma-linolenic acid
GLP-1	glucagon-like polypeptide-1
GMS	general medical services (GP) contract
γGT	γ-glutamyl transferase
HbA$_{1c}$	glycated haemoglobin
HBGM	home blood glucose monitoring
HD	haemodialysis
HDL	high density lipoprotein (cholesterol)
HHS	hyperosmolar hyperglycaemic state
HONK	hyperosmolar non-ketotic state
hsCRP	high-sensitivity CRP
i.v.	intravenous
ICA	islet-cell antibodies
IDF	International Diabetes Federation
IFG	impaired fasting glucose
IGT	impaired glucose tolerance
IHD	ischaemic heart disease
IRMA	intraretinal microvascular abnormality
ITU	intensive therapy unit
IVUS	intravascular ultrasound
LADA	latent autoimmune diabetes of the adult
LDL	low density lipoprotein (cholesterol)
LFT	liver function test
LH	luteinising hormone
LVH	left ventricular hypertrophy
MCV	mean cell volume
MI	myocardial infarction
MODY	maturity-onset diabetes of the young
m/r	modified release
MRI	magnetic resonance imaging
MRSA	methicillin-resistant *Staphylococcus aureus*
MSU	midstream urine
NAFLD	non-alcoholic fatty liver disease
NASH	non-alcoholic steatohepatitis
NGT	normal glucose tolerance
NICE	National Institute for Clinical Excellence
NIDDK	National Institute of Diabetes & Digestive Diseases & Kidney Diseases (USA)
NSTEMI	non-ST-segment elevation myocardial infarction
NVD	disc neovascularisation

NVE	new vessels elsewhere
OGTT	oral glucose tolerance test
OHA	oral hypoglycaemic agent
β-OHB	β-hydroxybutyrate
PAI-1	plasminogen activator inhibitor-1
PCI	percutaneous coronary intervention
PCOS	polycystic ovarian syndrome
PCT	primary care trust
PCU	progressive care unit (HDU, high-dependency unit)
PDE5	phosphodiesterase type 5 inhibitor
PEG	percutaneous endoscopic gastrostomy
PPAR	peroxisome proliferator-activated receptor
PSA	prostate-specific antigen
PTCA	percutaneous transluminal coronary angioplasty
PTH	parathyroid hormone
RBG	random blood glucose
RCT	randomised controlled trial
s.c.	subcutaneous
SNRI	selective norepinephrine (noradrenaline) reuptake inhibitor
SSRI	selective serotonin reuptake inhibitor
STEMI	ST-segment elevation myocardial infarction
T2DM	type 2 diabetes
TG	triglycerides
TIA	transient ischaemic attack
TZD	thiazolidinedione (glitazone, tee-zee-dee, USA)
ULN	upper limit of normal (laboratory range)
UTI	urinary tract infection
VEGF	vascular endothelial growth factor
WBC	white blood cell
WHO	World Health Organization

xiii

Studies and trials

Study name/ acronym	Full name of study	Year of publication	Brief description
4S*	Scandinavian Simvastatin Survival Study	1994	Secondary prevention with simvastatin 20–40 mg daily
AASK	African American Study of Kidney Disease and Hypertension	2002	Ramipril more effective than amlodipine or metoprolol in renal outcomes. No difference in intensive vs non-intensive BP reduction
ALLHAT	Antihypertensive and Lipid Lowering Treatment to Prevent Heart Attack	2002	Best first-line treatment for high-risk hypertensives (lisinopril, amlodipine, chlortalidone); primary (coronary) end point similar in all groups
ARBITER	Arterial Biology for the Investigation of the Treatment Effects of Reducing Cholesterol	2002	High-dose atorvastatin (80 mg daily) induced regression of atheroma (carotid IMT); stabilised by pravastatin 40 mg daily
ASCOT-LLA	Anglo-Scandinavian Cardiac Outcomes Trial – Lipid-Lowering Arm	2003	Reduction in major cardiovascular events in hypertensive subjects with atorvastatin 10 mg daily
ASCOT-BPLA	Anglo-Scandinavian Cardiac Outcomes Trial – Blood Pressure Lowering Arm	2005	Better BP lowering and cardiovascular outcomes in hypertensive patients treated with perindopril/amlodipine than atenolol/bendro-fluazide. Lower risk of new diabetes in non-diabetic subjects. Results broadly similar in diabetic patients
BARI	Bypass Angioplasty Revascularization Investigation	1996	Diabetic patients with multivessel disease had better outcomes with CABG compared with angioplasty (supported by more recent data)

Study name/ acronym	Full name of study	Year of publication	Brief description
BARI-2D*	BARI-Type 2 Diabetes	In progress	Coronary intervention + medical treatment vs. medical treatment only; insulin-sensitising regimen vs. insulin-replacing regimen (2x2 design)
BENEDICT*	Bergamo Nephrologic Diabetes Complications Trial	2004	Trandolapril and trandolapril/verapamil reduced progression to microalbuminuria in normoalbuminuric hypertensive type 2 diabetes patients (verapamil same as placebo)
BIP	Bezafibrate Infarction Prevention	2000	Secondary prevention. Non-significant reduction in events with bezafibrate in diabetic and non-diabetic patients
CALM*	Candesartan And Lisinopril Micro-albuminuria Study	2000	Candesartan 16 mg daily, lisinopril 20 mg daily or both in hypertensive microalbuminuric patients. Better BP reduction and reduction in alb:cr ratio with combination compared with either treatment alone
CALM II*	Candesartan And Lisinopril Micro-albuminuria Study II	2005	Candesartan 16 mg daily + lisinopril 20 mg daily showed no BP or proteinuria-lowering benefit over lisinopril 40 mg daily in micro/macroalbuminuric type 2 patients
CARDS*	Collaborative Atorvastatin Diabetes Study	2004	Primary prevention in type 2 diabetes. Atorvastatin 10 mg daily reduced all and serious CV events and stroke; borderline significant effect on all-cause mortality (RRR 25–40%)

Study name/ acronym	Full name of study	Year of publication	Brief description
CARE*	Cholesterol And Recurrent Events	1996	Secondary prevention with pravastatin 40 mg daily
CLAS	Cholesterol Lowering Atherosclerosis Study	1987	Early study showing beneficial effects of combination colestipol and niacin treatment on atheroma regression and coronary bypass grafts
CREATE-ECLA International GIK Study	Clinical Trial of Reviparin and Metabolic Modulation in Acute Myocardial Infarction Treatment Evaluation – Estudios Cardiologicas Latin American Study Group	2005	High dose insulin and glucose infusion for 24 hours had no effect at 30 days on death, non-fatal MI or reinfarction in STEMI (similar lack of effect in the ~3500 T2DM patients included in the study)
Da Qing		1997	Diet, exercise and diet + exercise reduced risk of progression of IGT to T2DM by 30-45% (no difference between interventions)
DAIS*	Diabetes Atherosclerosis Intervention Study	2001	Angiographic study of fenofibrate vs placebo in T2DM patients with ≥1 coronary lesion. Decreased progression and increased regression of lesions
DCCT*	Diabetes Control and Complications Trial	1993	T1DM. Improved glycaemic control decreased incidence and progression of micro-vascular complications
DETAIL*	Diabetics Exposed to Telmisartan And Enalapril	2004	T2DM with varying levels of micro- and macro-albuminuria. No difference in outcomes (GFR, BP, U Alb) on telmisartan 80 mg daily and enalapril 20 mg daily. Too few CV events to evaluate differences

xvi

Study name/ acronym	Full name of study	Year of publication	Brief description
DIABETES*	Diabetes and Sirolimus-Eluting Stent Trial	2005	Insulin and non-insulin treated patients had a lower 9-month restenosis, lumen loss, target-lesion revascularisation, and major adverse cardiac event rate when sirolimus-eluting stents were used compared with standard metal stents
DIGAMI*	Diabetes Mellitus Insulin-Glucose Infusion in Acute Myocardial Infarction Study	1997	MI patients with admission glucose >11 mmol/L, treated with GIK infusion, followed by sc insulin for at least 3 months decreased fatal, but not total reinfarctions over 3 years
DIRECT*	The Diabetic Retinopathy Candesartan Trial	2002 (trial design). Not yet reported	Effect of candesartan 16–32 mg daily on primary prevention of retinopathy in T1DM and primary and secondary prevention of retinopathy in T2DM, plus effect on albuminuria
DPP	EURODIAB Controlled Trial of Lisinopril in Insulin-Dependent Diabetes Mellitus	1997	Lisinopril in normotensive type 1 patients with normo- or microalbuminuria. Possible reduction in progression of retinopathy
EURODIAB*	European Community Concerted Action Programme in Diabetes	1989 onwards, continuing	IDDM Complications Study. Extended epidemiological study of type 1 diabetes throughout Europe
EUROPA	European Trial on Reduction of Cardiac Events with Perindopril in Stable Coronary Artery Disease	2003	Secondary prevention: perindopril 8 mg daily reduced risk of cardiovascular events by 20%; similar effect (not statistically significant) in diabetic substudy (PERSUADE, 2005)

Study name/ acronym	Full name of study	Year of publication	Brief description
FIELD*	Fenofibrate Inter-vention and Event Lowering in Diabetes	2005	Primary cardiac prevention in type 2 patients using a fibric acid drug
Finnish Diabetes Prevention Study		2001	Lifestyle intervention reduced risk of progression from IGT to T2DM by 60% over 3 years
GEMINI*	Glycemic Effects in Diabetes Mellitus: Carvedilol-Metoprolol Comparison in Hypertensives	2004	Neutral glycaemic effect of carvedilol (6.25–25 mg daily) and reduction in progression to microalbuminuria in hypertensive type 2 patients compared with metoprolol (50–200 mg daily)
GISSI-Prevenzione	Gruppo Italiano per lo Studio della Sopra-vvivenza nell'Infarto Miocardico	1999	1g n-3 polyunsaturated fish oils reduced risk of cardiovascular events and death post-MI by ~10–20%
HATS	HDL Atherosclerosis Treatment Study	2001	Niacin + simvastatin (but not antioxidants) reduced progression of coronary artery disease and tended to reduce CV end points in patients with normal LDL, but low HDL levels
HOPE*	Heart Outcomes Prevention Evaluation	2000	High-risk patients. Ramipril 10 mg daily for about 5 years reduced risk of CV events by ~20%, and reduced new-onset diabetes. Effects in diabetic patients very similar
HOPE-TOO	HOPE – The Ongoing Outcomes	2005	2.5 year observational study following HOPE. Continuing long-term CV benefit in original ramipril-treated group (apart from stroke). Overall 30% reduction in new-onset diabetes

Study name/ acronym	Full name of study	Year of publication	Brief description
HPS*	Heart Protection Study	2003	~25% reduction in cardiovascular events in type 2 patients over 5 years (simvastatin 40 mg daily). Type 1 patients and those with starting LDL <3 mmol/L benefited to same extent
IDNT*	Irbesartan Diabetes Nephropathy Trial		Type 2 patients with overt nephropathy; lower rate of progression to hard renal end points with irbesartan vs amlodipine, despite similar BP reduction
IRMA2*	Irbesartan Microalbuminuria II Trial	2001	Type 2 patients with microalbuminuria. Irbesartan 300 mg daily reduced risk of progression to proteinuria more than irbesartan 150 mg daily
ISAR- DIABETES*	Intracoronary Stenting and Angiographic Results – Do Diabetes Patients Derive Similar Benefits from Paclitaxel-Eluting and Sirolimus-Eluting Stents	2005	Sirolimus-eluting stents carry a lower risk of in-stent restenosis in diabetic (and non-diabetic) patients than paclitaxel-eluting stents
LIFE	The Losartan Intervention For Endpoint Reduction in Hypertension Study	2002	Patients with ECG evidence of LVH. Risk of CV end points reduced by ~25%. Total mortality risk in diabetic but not non-diabetic patients reduced by 40%
LIPID	Long-term Intervention with Pravastatin in Ischemic Disease	1998	Secondary prevention with pravastatin 40 mg daily

Study name/ acronym	Full name of study	Year of publication	Brief description
PEACE	Prevention of Events with Angiotensin Converting Enzyme Inhibition	2004	No significant benefit of trandolapril (up to 4 mg daily) on cardiovascular outcomes in patients with stable coronary artery disease (considered low-risk in comparison with HOPE patients)
PROACTIVE*	Prospective Pioglitazone Clinical Trial in Macrovascular Events	2005	Secondary prevention study in type 2 patients using proglitazone up to 45 mg daily added to any existing medication. Significant 16% RRR in all cause mortality/non-fatal MI/stroke after 2.8 years follow-up
PROVE-IT	Pravastatin or Atorvastatin Evaluation and Infection Therapy	2004	16% risk reduction in composite cardiac end points with atorvastatin 80 mg daily (median LDL 1.6 mmol/L) compared with pravastatin 40 mg daily (LDL 2.5 mmol/L) in patients with recent ACS
RENAAL*	Reduction of Endpoints in NIDDM with the Angiotensin II Antagonist Losartan	2001	Proteinuric type 2 patients with impaired renal function, treated with losartan 100 mg daily. Decreased risk of doubling serum creatinine and ESRF, but no effect on mortality or CV outcomes
REVERSAL	Reversal of Athero-sclerosis with Aggressive Lipid Lowering	2004	IVUS study comparing pravastatin 40 mg daily (atheroma progressed) with atorvastatin 80 mg daily (atheroma stabilised)

Study name/ acronym	Full name of study	Year of publication	Brief description
RIO-Europe/ lipids/North America	Rimonabant In Obesity	2005	Series of studies. Rimonabant 20 mg daily for 1 year reduced weight in overweight/obese patients by ~7 kg, and ameliorated many aspects of (and reduced progression to) the metabolic syndrome
SIRIUS*	Sirolimus-coated Bx velocity balloon-expandable stent	2004	Target lesion revascularisation significantly reduced in diabetic patients compared with bare metal stents (similar result in non-diabetic patients, but lower risk of repeat intervention)
Steno Type 2*		2003	T2DM with micro-albuminuria. Multifactorial intensive input (behaviour, glycaemic control, BP, dyslipidaemia, micro-albuminuria) reduced risk of CV disease, nephropathy, retinopathy, and autonomic neuropathy over 8 years
STOP-NIDDM	Study To Prevent NIDDM	2002	Acarbose 100 mg tds in IGT patients reduced risk of progression to diabetes by 25%, and also (controversially) risk of hypertension and CV events
TNT	Treating to New Targets	2005	High dose atorvastatin (80 mg daily) reduced risk of cardiovascular events by 22% compared with low dose (10 mg daily) in patients with stable coronary disease, but higher rates of adverse events, including ↑LFTs

Study name/ acronym	Full name of study	Year of publication	Brief description
TRIPOD		2002	50% reduction in progression from post-GDM IGT to type 2 diabetes with troglitazone. Terminated early
UKPDS*	United Kingdom Prospective Diabetes Study	1998	Intensive vs routine glycaemic and BP treatment in newly-diagnosed type 2 diabetes
VA CSDM*	Veterans Administration Cooperative Study on Glycemic Control and Complications in Type II Diabetes	1996	Pilot study, proof of concept similar to DCCT; maintenance of glycaemic control (intensive vs conventional)
VADT*	Veterans Administration Diabetes Trial	2010?	Full RCT follow-on from VA CSDM. Improved glycaemic control and macrovascular events
VA-HIT	Veterans Affairs Cooperative Studies Program HDL-C Intervention Trial	1999	Secondary prevention in patients with low LDL, but mild insulin-resistant dyslipidaemia, using gemfibrozil (no effect on LDL) over 5 years. 24% risk reduction in diabetic patients; effect most marked in the most hyperinsulinaemic subjects
XENDOS		2004	50% reduction in progression of IGT (but not NGT) to type 2 diabetes with orlistat 120 mg tds for 4 years

*Studies either in diabetic patients exclusively, or where results in diabetic patients have been reported separately

xxii

1 CLASSIFICATION AND DIAGNOSIS

The history of the classification and chemical diagnosis of diabetes is long and complex, with occasional hints of American-European tension. The revised classification proposed in 1997 by the American Diabetes Association (ADA) has been generally agreed in the World Health Organization (WHO) report of 1999, as was the major change to lower the diagnostic criterion for diabetes from a fasting venous plasma glucose (FPG) of ≥7.8 to ≥7.0 mmol/L. The epidemiological evidence for the lower level was solid – the incidence of microvascular complications (retinopathy), very low (but not, probably, zero) at FPG below 7.0, rises rapidly above this threshold. Normal FPG was until recently considered to be ≤6.0 mmol/L, but there was a widespread consensus that this was too high, and the most recent definition of normal glucose (ADA, International Diabetes Federation, IDF) is ≤5.5 mmol/L (see below and Chapter 2).

The ADA proposal to abandon the oral glucose tolerance test (OGTT) and to classify all states using fasting glucose levels was met with less universal agreement, because the 2-hour blood glucose level in the standard 75 g OGTT is epidemiologically more strongly associated with cardiovascular endpoints than the fasting value and may yield higher diagnostic rates in certain groups, for example the elderly, the non-obese and SE Asians. In addition, although fasting and 2-hour glucose levels are strongly correlated in epidemiological studies, this may not be the case in an individual patient. The OGTT is therefore recommended when there is diagnostic doubt – persistent FPG levels in the impaired fasting glucose (IFG) range (5.6–6.9 mmol/L).

While this scheme is complex and difficult for the non-specialist to remember, it is extremely valuable. Nearly all patients can be classified using fasting venous plasma glucose levels together with the OGTT in a specified group of patients – more than ever there is now no justification for terms like 'borderline', 'potential', 'slightly elevated', etc. Because of the adverse cardiovascular impact of impaired glucose tolerance, every attempt should be made to come to a definitive diagnosis.

Classification

The 1997 ADA scheme has tried to use pathophysiology rather than treatment for classification purposes. The terms 'insulin-dependent' and 'non-insulin-dependent' have been replaced by 'type 1' and 'type 2' (a point of detail is the use of Arabic, not Roman numerals). However, in practice, hybrid terminology still persists, e.g. 'insulin-treated type 2 diabetes', since treatment modality remains important to clinicians and to patients.

Other terms that are now obsolete, but still appear to be in widespread use are shown in Table 1.1.

Table 1.1   Obsolete terms for type 1 and 2 diabetes

Type 1	Type 2
Type I	Type II
Juvenile-onset	Adult-onset, maturity-onset
IDDM	NIDDM
Insulin-dependent	Non-insulin-dependent

Type 1 diabetes (β-cell destruction, usually leading to complete insulin deficiency)

Operational definition
* Acute onset under the age of 30 in a non-obese person (but see important provisos below).
* Ketonuria and/or metabolic acidosis at presentation.
* Immediate and permanent requirement for insulin (though insulin requirements may be minimal during the honeymoon period – 6–18 months after diagnosis).
* No evidence of microvascular complications at presentation.

Note
* Type 1 diabetes can occur at any age, early childhood to old age, but classical type 1 diabetes has a peak incidence in pre-school children (age 4–6 years) and around puberty (11–16, earlier peak in girls than boys); there is a pronounced seasonal variation, most cases occurring between autumn and spring. There is a consistent slight preponderance of cases in males.

- Lower, constant incidence after this age, with a hint of a slight peak in the late 30s.
- Incidence is steadily increasing, especially rapidly in the under 5s.
- The 'Accelerator Hypothesis' postulates that β-cell loss is accelerated under the influence of insulin resistance, epidemiologically being fuelled by the obesity epidemic. One of its predictions, that the age at diagnosis of type 1 diabetes is inversely related to body mass index (BMI), has been confirmed in several studies.
- Risk of type 1 diabetes in offspring of type 1 diabetic parents is widely reported to be higher in offspring of type 1 diabetic fathers (5–9%) than in offspring of diabetic mothers (2–3%).

Serological markers of islet-cell destruction are:

- insulin antibodies (obsolete)
- islet-cell antibodies (ICA)
- antibodies to glutamic acid decarboxylase (GAD_{65})
- antibodies to the tyrosine phosphatases IA-2 and IA-2β.

Testing for combinations of these antibodies increases their power to predict type 1 diabetes, and also increases diagnostic accuracy. Only ICA and GAD antibodies are widely available, and they should be requested only if there is a clinical dilemma – for example, to confirm whether newly diagnosed diabetes without ketonuria or acidosis in a non-obese middle-aged person is late-onset type 1 diabetes, or, more commonly, to distinguish between type 1 and type 2 diabetes in adolescence – but even these tests are not completely reliable, and must not substitute for careful clinical supervision and frequent review where there is uncertainty.

Endocrine diseases associated with type 1 diabetes

There are two forms of autoimmune polyglandular syndrome (APS) associated with type 1 diabetes. The rare type 1 APS consists of mucocutaneous candidiasis with nail dystrophy, hypoparathyroidism and Addison's disease (no female preponderance). Type 1 diabetes occurs in 2–12% of patients. The much more common type 2 APS, occurring predominantly in females who are HLA DR3/4 positive, consists of, in order of decreasing frequency:

- Addison's disease
- autoimmune thyroid disease (usually Hashimoto's thyroiditis, but sometimes Graves' disease)

- type 1 diabetes
- primary gonadal failure
- less common associations: alopecia, vitiligo, pernicious anaemia, hypophysitis, coeliac disease, myasthenia gravis, primary biliary cirrhosis.

The syndrome, however, does not represent the commonest associations in practice. Autoimmune thyroid disease is common in type 1 diabetes, and patients should be regularly screened, perhaps annually, with a TSH measurement (a baseline anti-thyroid peroxidase antibody measurement would be wise). Coeliac disease is much more common than previously thought. About 2–6% of type 1 patients have serological evidence of coeliac disease, and many units screen newly diagnosed type 1 patients for antibodies to tissue transglutaminase, currently the most reliable marker. Schmidt's syndrome is autoimmune Addison's disease + autoimmune hypothyroidism (± type 1 diabetes) and, like many eponyms, is unnecessarily confusing in an already difficult area.

Type 2 diabetes (hyperinsulinaemia, insulin resistance, and variable insulin deficiency or secretory defect, all of which are detectable at diagnosis)

Type 2 diabetes is usually not difficult to diagnose and shows the following features:

- onset of osmotic symptoms over a variable period – weeks to years – in an overweight middle-aged person (mean BMI at onset around 28)
- variable degree of weight loss
- ketonuria minimal or absent
- positive family history in first-degree relatives is common
- pre-diagnosis duration of hyperglycaemia is 7–10 years or more, with perhaps another 10 years of the metabolic syndrome preceding this, so approximately 20% have detectable complications at presentation. Some may present with clinically advanced complications (e.g. acute macrovascular event – stroke or myocardial infarction (MI) – or microvascular complications – visual loss from advanced retinopathy, neuropathic foot ulceration, stick-positive proteinuria or frank nephropathy).

In clinical practice, there is now considerable difficulty in classifying some patients, particularly at onset. Examples are as follows.

Late-onset type 1 diabetes

Also known as latent autoimmune diabetes of the adult (LADA), late-onset type 1 diabetes is increasingly recognised. Nearly 12% of patients recruited to the UKPDS had antibodies to at least one islet-cell antigen, and this rate is consistent with other studies. Always be vigilant for ketonuria, and be aware of the subtle phenotype. Features are:

- usual onset in the 40s
- patients are usually only moderately overweight (e.g. BMI 27) and less likely to have features of the metabolic syndrome
- poor and/or short-lived response to oral hypoglycaemic agents, especially sulphonylureas. In the UKPDS cohort, 60% of antibody-positive patients required insulin treatment within 2 years of diagnosis, compared with 15% of antibody-negative patients
- high incidence of coexistent autoimmune diseases, especially hypothyroidism
- diagnosis can be made definitively by finding positive anti-GAD antibodies.

Type 2 diabetes presenting as diabetic ketoacidosis ('Flatbush' diabetes)

This type of diabetes, first reported in obese African-American men, usually in their 30s, is now commonly seen in the UK in African and African-Caribbean people. It presents with classical, sometimes severe, diabetic ketoacidosis.

After discharge on insulin, doses rapidly fall, often over 3–6 months, or even less, and patients are eventually controlled on oral hypoglycaemics or even diet alone. Complete remission – good control on diet alone – occurs in 30–40% of these patients, and may last for more than 3 years. Recurrence of diabetic ketoacidosis is recognised, but clinically rare. Flatbush diabetes is negative for autoimmune markers for type 1 diabetes: the pathogenesis is unclear, but is presumably related to partial, temporary, β-cell failure.

Type 2 diabetes in obese children and adolescents

This was first recognised in the early 1980s in the USA, but with increasing frequency in the 1990s. Most are obese ethnic minority patients (especially African-Americans, but also Hispanic Americans and native Americans). Ketosis and ketoacidosis are much more common in ethnic minority patients than in white patients, though, as with the adults, they are ICA negative. In Japan, where type 1 diabetes is rare, type 2 diabetes is the most common form of diabetes in adolescence. Long-term follow-up in small numbers of North American patients confirms a very high rate of microvascular complications and pregnancy loss. They are also very likely to develop premature macrovascular complications. There are no UK screening recommendations, but the ADA recommends that overweight children (>85th percentile for age and sex) aged ≥10 years should have fasting glucose tested every 2 years in the presence of any two of the following risk factors:

- family history of type 2 diabetes (first- or second-degree relatives)
- race/ethnicity (in UK: South Asian, African and African-Caribbean origin)
- features of insulin resistance: acanthosis nigricans (probably the most important clinical feature), dyslipidaemia, hypertension, polycystic ovarian syndrome (PCOS).

Despite the increasing likelihood of patients presenting with ketosis and/or acidosis being truly type 2 patients, from the point of view of safe management, they should all be managed initially with insulin, with very careful diabetes team follow-up (see Chapter 3).

Other specific types

- Genetic defects of β-cell function, e.g. mitochondrial DNA – maternally inherited diabetes and deafness; maturity-onset diabetes of the young (MODY). Six types are currently described: MODY2 (glucokinase mutation, ~20% of cases), MODY1 and MODY3–6 (transcription-factor mutations, the more common, HNF1α, comprising about 60% of cases).
- Genetic defects in insulin action, e.g. lipoatrophic diabetes, Rabson–Mendenhall syndrome, leprechaunism.
- Diseases of the exocrine pancreas, e.g. pancreatitis, pancreatic carcinoma, cystic fibrosis, haemochromatosis, fibrocalculous pancreatopathy. These processes cause more destruction of the glucagon-producing α-cells than does autoimmune type 1 diabetes. Since glucagon excess is a major pathophysiological feature of DKA, these patients are less prone to DKA than type 1 patients (see Chapter 3). Patients >50 years old with recent-onset type 2 diabetes have an approximately eightfold increased risk of pancreatic

cancer, by which time the disease is usually advanced; interestingly, the diabetes is serologically mediated through insulin resistance, and not pancreatic β-cell destruction.

- Endocrinopathies associated with hormones mediating insulin resistance, e.g. acromegaly (growth hormone), Cushing's syndrome (cortisol), phaeochromocytoma (catecholamines, especially noradrenaline), glucagonoma. Cushing's disease or syndrome may be present in up to 5% of obese, poorly controlled (HbA$_{1c}$ >8%) type 2 patients but this finding is difficult to translate into clinical practice, especially considering the phenotypical overlap with the polycystic ovarian syndrome, which is extremely common in women with type 2 diabetes.
- Drug- or chemical-induced, e.g. glucocorticoids (see Chapter 4), high-dose thiazides, β-blockers, protease inhibitors, some of the second-generation antipsychotics (especially olanzapine and clozapine (see Chapter 2), calcineurin inhibitors (ciclosporin, tacrolimus) contributing to the recently described syndrome of new-onset diabetes after transplantation.
- Infections, e.g. rubella, cytomegalovirus.
- Uncommon forms of immune-mediated diabetes, e.g. stiff man (properly, stiff person) syndrome, associated with high GAD$_{65}$ antibody levels; anti-insulin receptor antibodies.
- Other genetic syndromes sometimes associated with diabetes, e.g. Turner's syndrome (markedly increased risk of both type 1 and type 2 diabetes), Klinefelter's syndrome, Friedrich's ataxia, Huntington's chorea, myotonic dystrophy.

Gestational diabetes mellitus (GDM)

Any degree of glucose intolerance with onset or first recognition during pregnancy is diagnosed as GDM. The diagnosis is independent of treatment modality (diet alone or diet with insulin).

Diagnosis

The chemical diagnosis of diabetes is currently based on FPG values (fasting = no caloric intake for at least 8 hours); whole blood and capillary blood values are no longer quoted. The 2-hour post-75 g glucose load value is retained for the diagnosis of impaired glucose tolerance (and isolated post-challenge hyperglycaemia).

In the presence of classical symptoms

- Random plasma glucose ≥11.1 mmol/L – no further tests are required.
- Casual plasma glucose 5.5–11.0 mmol/L – confirmatory FPG is required.

Without classical symptoms

Table 1.2 Diagnosis of diabetes without classical symptoms

	FPG (mmol/L)	Comment
Normal	≤5.5	Mean FPG in a lean population is around 4
IFG	5.6–6.9	Repeated levels in this range → OGTT for confirmation of glycaemic state
Diabetes	≥7.0	

Use of HbA$_{1c}$

At present glycated haemoglobin (HbA$_{1c}$) measurements cannot be used reliably on their own to diagnose diabetes. International agreement on HbA$_{1c}$ measurements has now been reached. Implementing the change worldwide is a formidable challenge, but once achieved, the role of HbA$_{1c}$ as the sole indicator of diabetes is likely to become established. At present, however, HbA$_{1c}$, together with blood glucose measurements, is often helpful in the practical setting, for example:

- patients who have deliberately lost weight on the recognition of diabetic symptoms, and who present with normal fasting glucose levels. An elevated HbA$_{1c}$ would indicate prolonged preceding hyperglycaemia
- in-patients with elevated random glucose levels in association with an intercurrent illness, where a glucose tolerance test would be impractical or unreliable
- where patients decline an OGTT despite repeated fasting glucose measurements in the range 5.6–6.9 mmol/L.

An HbA$_{1c}$ >6.0% would be widely regarded as abnormal.

OGTT interpretation

Table 1.3   OGTT interpretation

	Fasting	2-h	Significance/comments
Normal	<5.6	<7.8	If there are symptoms suggesting diabetes, then consider other causes
IFG	5.6–6.9	<7.8	Not known; not normal, but not as strong an association with ↑risk of IHD as IGT
IGT	<5.6	7.8–11.1	See below
IFG + IGT	5.6–6.9	7.8–11.1	Very high risk of progression to diabetes; effectively treat as diabetes
Diabetes	≥7.0	≥11.1	The diagnosis of diabetes is based on EITHER the fasting OR the 2-h value, so diabetes may exist with normal fasting levels, i.e. <7.0 (but a 2-h level ≥11.1, so-called isolated post-challenge hyperglycaemia). This false-negative rate is around 3%

Impaired glucose tolerance (IGT)

People with IGT are usually normoglycaemic on casual testing, and it can be diagnosed only on an OGTT. IGT clusters with the other components of the metabolic syndrome (see Chapter 2). Because of this, it is a high-risk state for coronary heart disease, and without intervention around 6% of patients with IGT will progress to type 2 diabetes every year. Since 1997, six studies on prevention of progression have reported; three (STOP-NIDDM, 2002; TRIPOD 2002; XENDOS, 2004) used pharmacological interventions (acarbose, troglitazone and orlistat respectively), while two employed intensive lifestyle interventions to reduce weight and increase exercise (Da Qing, 1997; Finnish Diabetes Prevention Study, 1997). The Diabetes Prevention Program (2002) had both a lifestyle and and a pharmacological (metformin) arm, lifestyle interventions being more effective than metformin (risk reduction 60 vs. 30% over about 3 years).

Practical implications
- When detected, IGT and its associated features of insulin resistance should all be actively managed.
- Multimodal management is likely to be of maximum value in the routine clinical setting, i.e. dietetic intervention to reduce weight by 4–6 kg, increase exercise to 150 min per week, and addition of either metformin 850 mg b.d. or acarbose, increasing if tolerated to 100 mg t.d.s.
- The glitazones are likely to be of value, but they cannot yet be recommended; troglitazone was withdrawn from the Diabetes Prevention Program in 1998, though over a short period it was at least as effective as the other interventions. The newer agents rosiglitazone and pioglitazone (see Chapter 7) have not yet been formally tested in this setting; clinical trials are in progress.

Screening for diabetes

Value and strategy are not defined in the UK, and firm recommendations are unlikely to be made for a year or two. However, the American Diabetes Association/National Institutes of Health have made the following preliminary recommendations for screening/diabetes prevention on the basis of the Diabetes Prevention Program. They suggest that primary care providers should screen, using fasting plasma glucose:

- all people ≥45 years of age, especially those with BMI ≥25 (a more practical proposal might be to screen initially those with BMI ≥30, who have an ~20× increased risk compared with those of BMI <20; a BMI ≥40 carries ~40× increased risk)
- people ≤45 years + BMI ≥25 (or ≥30) or additional diabetes risk factor:
  - first-degree family history of diabetes (parents and siblings)
  - previous gestational diabetes – a very important group for screening. Around 5% of diet-treated white GDM patients progress each year to type 2 diabetes, about 10× the background rate. The rate is increasing with increasing population obesity. Obese, ethnic minority patients with post-partum IGT constitute the very highest risk group, especially for development of premature coronary heart disease, and annual screening would seem prudent, though not yet officially recommended

10

- hypertension (two- to threefold increased risk)
- dyslipidaemia
- ethnic minority.

See above for recommendations on screening younger people.

Further recommendations (ADA/NIDDK)

- Rescreen all normoglycaemic individuals every 3 years.
- Counsel all patients with IFG or IGT to lose 5–10% of body weight + exercise 30 min/day.
- Test all patients with IFG/IGT every 1–2 years for development of diabetes.

2 THE METABOLIC SYNDROME

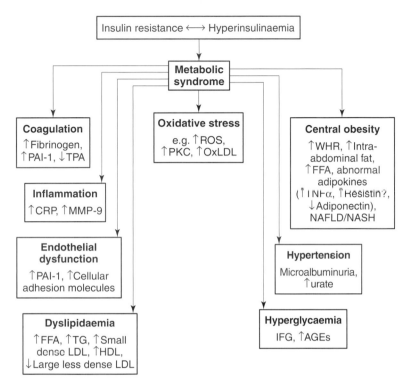

Figure 2.1 Some clinical and laboratory features of the metabolic syndrome. AGEs, advanced glycation end products; CRP, C-reactive protein; FFA, free fatty acids; IFG, impaired fasting glucose; MMP-9, matrix metalloproteinase 9; NAFLD/NASH, non-alcoholic fatty liver disease/non-alcoholic steatohepatitis; OxLDL, oxidised LDL; PAI-1, plasminogen activator inhibitor 1; PKC, protein kinase C; ROS, reactive oxygen species; TNF-α, tumour necrosis factor alpha; TPA, tissue plasminogen activator; WHR, waist-hip ratio.

Type 2 diabetes cannot be understood, or its management optimised, without an understanding of the metabolic syndrome. Its first description as syndrome 'X', in 1998, by Gerald Reaven, is now complemented by a preliminary understanding of its mechanistic basis, insulin resistance.

Table 2.1 Criteria for definition of metabolic syndrome

	ATP III	WHO	AACE	IDF
Obesity	Waist circumference: >102 cm (men), 94–102 if other risk factors; >88 cm (women)	BMI >30 kg/m2 and/ or W:H ratio >0.95 (men), >0.85 (women)	BMI ≥25 kg/m2	Waist circumference: Europid, ≥94 cm (men), ≥80 cm (female)*
Blood pressure (mmHg)	≥130/≥85	≥140/≥90 and/or antihypertensive medication	≥135/≥85	≥130/≥85 or treatment or previously diagnosed hypertension
Triglycerides	≥1.7 mm/L	≥1.7mmol/L	≥1.7 mmol/L	≥1.7 mmol/L (or specific treatment for this abnormality)
HDL cholesterol (mmol/L)	<1.0 (men), <1.3 (women)	<0.9 (men), <1.0 (women)	<1.0 (men), <1.3 (women)	<1.03 (men), <1.29 (women) or specific treatment

Glycaemia/ insulin resistance	FPG ≥6.1 mmol/L (recent suggestion ≥5.5)	Insulin resistance; type 2 diabetes; IFG/IGT; low glucose uptake (below lowest quartile using hyperinsulinaemic, euglycaemic conditions)	FPG 6.1–6.9 mmol/L; 2-h post-glucose challenge >7.8 mmol/L	FPG ≥5.6 or pre-existing diabetes
Others	Urinary albumin excretion ≥20 µg/min or albumin:creatinine ratio ≥30 mg/g		Family history type 2 diabetes mellitus (DM), ↑BP or CVD; PCOS; sedentary lifestyle; advancing age; ethnic group with high risk for type 2 DM or CVD	
Definition	≥3 factors	Insulin resistance + 2 other risk factors	Clinical judgement	Central obesity + 2 other risk factors

*Waist measurement criteria differ according to ethnic group, wherever they have emigrated to: South Asian (Chinese, Malay, Asian-Indian), ≥90 cm (men), ≥80 cm (women); Japanese, ≥85 cm (men), ≥90 cm (women). The IDF recommends that European criteria should be used for sub-Saharan Africans and Eastern Mediterranean and Middle East (Arab) populations until more specific data are available.

The two terms are often used interchangeably, but the distinction should be made: insulin resistance is the failure of insulin to exert its major effect, facilitating glucose uptake in insulin-sensitive peripheral tissues – muscle, adipose tissue and liver. It is difficult to measure insulin resistance, even under strict laboratory conditions (hyperinsulinaemic euglycaemic clamp), and though simpler measures have been proposed, for example based on fasting measurements of insulin and glucose, these are still not routinely available. Instead, the phenotypic manifestations of the metabolic syndrome are used as a surrogate for insulin resistance. Several definitions have been proposed (National Cholesterol Education Program Adult Treatment Panel III [NCEP ATP III], WHO, AACE [American Association of Clinical Endocrinologists] and the most recent, IDF) but they all contain five core features:

- Central obesity: waist circumference, rather than body mass index, is the key measurement, because it correlates best with intra-abdominal fat mass, a major factor behind the pro-inflammatory adipokines thought to be driving the syndrome. Criterion values wobble somewhat (see below); the IDF values (≥94 cm [37 inches] for European males; ≥80 cm [31.5 inches] for females) are stringent, and the ATP values (102 cm, male; 88 cm, female) are probably more practical.
- Hypertriglyceridaemia: in clinical practice, the 'hypertriglyceridaemic waist' can identify with high reliability most subjects with the full syndrome – high waist circumference together with fasting triglyceride >2.0 mmol/L.
- Low HDL cholesterol: correlates closely with ↑TG.
- Hypertension: the WHO and IDF definitions include the use of antihypertensive medication.
- Hyperglycaemia: abnormal fasting glucose (impaired fasting glucose) is ≥5.6 mmol/L in the IDF definition. The WHO and IDF definitions include diagnosed type 2 diabetes (and IFG/IGT in WHO) in this category.

The significance of the metabolic syndrome

- In general, the more the features, the greater the degree of insulin resistance.
- It is an important risk factor for CHD, independent of the conventional risk factors; for example, type 2 patients who do not have the

metabolic syndrome (~20% of all type 2 patients) do not have significantly increased risk of CHD (this group of patients will clinically overlap with those who have late-onset type 1 diabetes, LADA).

- It is a major public health problem: in the USA 20–30% of Americans have NCEP-defined metabolic syndrome, rising to ~44% in those >50 years of age; Hispanic Americans have a higher prevalence, South-East Asians lower. In the UK, ~30% of South Asians (India, Pakistan, Bangladesh) have the metabolic syndrome, compared with ~16% of Europeans, and ~20% of African-Caribbeans (but note the impact of the slight increase in prevalence in this last group is not associated with increased CHD risk, partly accounted for by a favourable lipid profile; the same was thought to be a factor behind the so-called 'Hispanic paradox' in the USA, though this group probably does have a significantly higher risk of CHD).
- It is associated with increased rates of macrovascular complications in both type 1 and type 2 diabetes.

Clinical associations

The number of clinical associations continues to grow. Always consider the syndrome when patients present with the following. Remember that there is a significant proportion of lean metabolic syndrome patients ('metabolically obese, normal weight'), especially hypertensive, non-diabetic and PCOS patients:

- abdominal obesity
- polycystic ovarian syndrome
- hypertension
- any macrovascular event
- chronic kidney disease and microalbuminuria (independent of diabetes)
- sleep apnoea syndrome
- non-alcoholic fatty liver disease/non-alcoholic steatohepatitis (NAFLD/NASH)
- gout/hyperuricaemia; possible association with ↓serum phosphate
- mixed hyperlipidaemia, especially if there is a family history of CHD (familial combined hyperlipidaemia)
- erectile dysfunction is a likely association; the more the components of the metabolic syndrome the higher the prevalence

- second-generation antipsychotics. Patients taking clozapine and olanzapine have a higher risk of developing the metabolic syndrome compared with other agents, especially the newer drugs such as aripiprazole and ziprasidone. These drugs also increase the risk of type 2 diabetes (see Chapter 1). Risperidone and quetiapine are associated with weight gain, but the risks of diabetes and dyslipidaemia are probably lower.

Associations with laboratory measurements

These are also increasing in number, though not yet part of the definition of the syndrome. Examples are:

- inflammatory markers: high-sensitivity (hs) C-reactive protein (CRP) – the top candidate for inclusion in the syndrome
- other lipid measurements: hyperapolipoprotein B (hyperapo B – the sum of all the atherogenic lipoprotein classes) and small, dense LDL, forming an important metabolic triad together with hyperinsulinaemia
- coagulation: ↑fibrinogen, ↑PAI-1, ↓tPA (tissue plasminogen activator)
- oxidative stress: ↑oxidised LDL
- others: microalbuminuria in the absence of diabetes (>20 µg/min is included in the WHO definition of the metabolic syndrome, though cardiovascular risk is elevated in those with sub-criterion levels of microalbuminuria, and even at levels lower than the detection limit of routine assays).

Apart from microalbuminuria, hsCRP is the only measurement that is generally available.

Non-alcoholic fatty liver disease (NAFLD)

NAFLD is one of the most important manifestations of the metabolic syndrome. Up to 75% of type 2 patients have some form of fatty liver, the histological severity increasing with increasing ATP III score. There is increasing evidence that ~30% of patients with its more advanced form, non-alcoholic steatohepatitis (NASH) progress to fibrosis and cirrhosis; many patients with 'cryptogenic' cirrhosis are now thought to have progressed from NASH. The current definition allows alcohol up to 28 units a week (men), 14 units a week (women). Elevations of transaminases (AST, ALT) are usually mild, commonly <1.5× upper limit of reference range, i.e. <50 IU/L, and rarely >10×. ALT is usually >AST; the converse suggests significant fibrosis or cirrhosis. Iron indices, which are frequently elevated, but not to the level associated with genetic haemochromatosis, and hepatitis serology should be checked; most patients should have a liver ultrasound scan. Consider the possibility of autoimmune liver disease.

Management of the metabolic syndrome

Investigations

- Fasting glucose and full lipid screen; if FPG ≥5.6 mmol/L, proceed to formal diagnosis with an OGTT (see Chapter 1).
- Liver function tests: ALT, (AST), γGT, ALP.
- Serum urate.
- Measurement of urinary albumin excretion, either 24-hour urinary albumin, or albumin:creatinine ratio (though cardiovascular risk is already increasing at levels well below the detection limit of most laboratory assays, ~6 mg/24 h).
- Resting ECG.
- Where available: ferritin, fibrinogen, hsCRP, carotid artery ultrasound for common carotid intima-media thickness – a reliable non-invasive surrogate measure of cardiovascular risk.

Clinical management must be comprehensive:

- Weight loss (~7–10% of body weight, with a 500–1000 calorie/day reduction – DPP). Approximately 8 kg weight loss has been shown to reverse hepatic steatosis in type 2 diabetic patients.
- Smoking cessation advice.
- Increasing activity (regular bouts of 15–60 minutes exercise).
- Treating hypertension with metabolically neutral or beneficial drugs (ACE inhibitors/ARBs, calcium channel blockers).
- Low-dose aspirin in those with a calculated 10-year CVD risk ≥10%.

Metformin, orlistat or acarbose would be justified in patients with IGT (see Chapter 1). In the DPP, where about 50% of participants had the metabolic syndrome at baseline, metformin and lifestyle intervention reduced the risk of progression to the metabolic syndrome and, less markedly, increased resolution of the metabolic syndrome – but lifestyle interventions were uniformly more effective.

19

The management of the dyslipidaemia is difficult, because there is no epidemiological or clinical trial data in the absence of frank diabetes or established CHD, and since many of these patients are relatively young, any drug treatment might be long-term. Fibric acid drugs would be justified if TG is >5 mmol/L, on account of the risk of acute pancreatitis; if there is concomitant elevated LDL, statin treatment would again be justified if risk, formally assessed, was appropriately elevated (>15% 10-year risk).

New developments

The recently described endocannabinoid system has cannibinoid-1 (CB_1) receptors in several brain areas associated with appetite regulation, and also in peripheral tissues, including adipose tissue, liver and muscle. In a 12-month clinical trial (RIO-Europe, 2005), the CB_1 receptor blocker rimonabant, 20 mg daily, together with a hypocaloric diet (usually described as 'mildly' hypocaloric, but actually substantially so – ~600 kCal/day) reduced NCEP-ATP III-defined metabolic syndrome by about 50% in an obese (mean BMI 35) non-diabetic population. There were significant reductions in weight and waist circumference (mean 8 kg and 8 cm, respectively), TG, glucose (~0.1 mmol/L), insulin and insulin resistance, but no changes in BP, LDL or total cholesterol, or glucose tolerance status. HDL-cholesterol increased independently of weight loss. Rimonabant is likely to be important in the medical management of obesity-associated metabolic syndrome, though central effects, especially nausea, are quite frequent, and depression occurred in about 3% of patients. Its minor effect on glucose levels means that combination therapy would be needed in diabetes patients with the metabolic syndrome.

3 HYPERGLYCAEMIC EMERGENCIES AND HYPOGLYCAEMIA

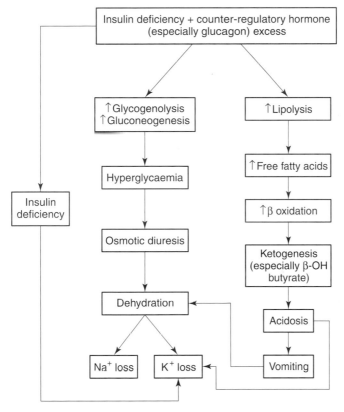

Figure 3.1 Pathophysiology of diabetic ketoacidosis.

The differentiation between diabetic ketoacidosis (DKA) and hyperosmolar hyperglycaemic state (HHS, formerly hyperosmolar non-ketotic state, 'HONK') is not difficult, but is important. HHS has a different pathogenesis, it occurs in a different group of patients (older, type 2, often with significant comorbidity), and carries a worse prognosis. Much of the excess mortality found in younger type 1 patients is due to DKA, though fortunately deaths due to DKA are very uncommon (EURODIAB), and currently certainly less than the 4–10% rate quoted in the literature. Nevertheless, both conditions require constant vigilance of the clinical state and biochemistry; neither is a 'set piece' emergency that can be run purely by protocol.

It is also important to make the distinction between DKA and hyperglycaemic states that require different, less urgent and less intensive treatment. It is easy to write 'DKA', because it is a simple acronym, but although it may seem simplistic, all elements must be present in order to make the diagnosis:

- hyperglycaemia – though it is not always very marked
- ketosis (signifying insulin deficiency)
- acidosis (rarely, alcohol intoxication or salicylate overdosage can present as ketoacidosis).

Therefore, it is important to distinguish DKA from:

- severe hyperglycaemia – poorly controlled diabetes (many type 1 patients occasionally have blood glucose levels >20 mmol/L without ketosis or acidosis; conversely, note there is no threshold of blood glucose level below which DKA can be excluded)
- ketosis – high blood glucose levels with ketonuria (≥1+) but no acidosis in an otherwise well patient. Significant ketonuria is much less common than it used to be in out-patient practice; always try to find a reason for it, and ensure that the patient has a supply of urine sticks for detection of ketones (e.g. Ketostix, Bayer; Ketur Test, Roche Diagnostics) so that they can monitor the ketonuria, and ensure that it remits within 12–24 hours – they must report back if it does not.

Precipitating factors

- Newly presenting type 1 or type 2 diabetes (10–20%)
- Infection, most commonly chest, urinary tract or gastrointestinal (30–40%)
- Other intercurrent medical illness, e.g. myocardial infarction, stroke, occasionally surgical illness

Table 3.1 Clinical features of DKA and HHS

	DKA	HHS
Patients	Type 1 diabetes (but see Chapter 1 for important exceptions)	Type 2 diabetes
Duration of history	Short, often <24 h	Longer, several days, sometimes insidious
Pathogenesis	Insulin deficiency Glucagon (and other counter-regulatory hormone) excess Renal impairment Reduced thirst	Insulin deficiency Abnormal metabolism of non-esterified fatty acids
Mortality rate	<4%	20–30%
Complications	Cerebral oedema (especially in the young) Respiratory distress syndrome Thromboembolism Rhabdomyolysis	Thromboembolism
Working biochemical definition	Arterial pH <7.3 Arterial bicarbonate ≤15 mmol/L (in early compensated stages, bicarbonate buffers ketoacids, so [HCO$_3^-$] is low but pH normal)* Urinary ketones ≥2+	Arterial pH >7.3 Plasma osmolality† >320 mosmol/kg Plasma bicarbonate >18 mmol/L

*In DKA there is an anion gap ([Na$^+$ + K$^+$] – [HCO$_3^-$ + Cl$^-$]), even in the absence of lipaemia or ethanol – probably due to acetone, decreased plasma water fraction, amino acids and glycerol. Normal anion gap is 7–9 mmol/L; the measurement in increased anion gap acidosis is >10–12 mmol/L.
†Plasma osmolality = 2[Na$^+$] + 2[K$^+$] + [urea] + [glucose]: normal value 280–300 mosmol/L. Calculated osmolality may seriously underestimate the true value. Plasma osmolality correlates with level of mental obtundation in both DKA and HHS.

- Omission of insulin (13–30%):
  - most commonly through not implementing the 'sick day' rule not to stop insulin treatment if the patient is not eating ('no food, no insulin')

- accidental, e.g. failure of subcutaneous insulin infusion pump
- Other causes: 'brittle diabetes'; patients with advanced neuropathy and gastroparesis, leading to recurrent vomiting; the antipsychotic drugs olanzapine and clozapine are associated with DKA, probably through a direct inhibitory effect on insulin secretion.

A common clinical scenario is the young person with type 1 diabetes who drinks too much alcohol at a party, vomits, and fails to take their bedtime insulin and mealtime insulin the following morning and lunchtime. In up to 40% of cases, there is no identifiable precipitating factor.

Table 3.2 Symptoms and signs of DKA and HHS

Symptoms	Signs
Osmotic (polydipsia, polyuria, weight loss)	Dehydration
HHS often exacerbated by consuming large quantities of sugar-containing drinks	Drowsiness, coma (uncommon nowadays – consider other causes, e.g. alcohol, drugs, and CT scan-detectable causes such as stroke and head injury)
Malaise → obtundation	Hypotension and vasodilatation (acidosis)

Abdominal pain. Contributory factors:
    Delayed gastric emptying
    Ileus-induced acidosis
    Ketosis itself
	Ketones on breath (not everyone can smell them)
	Kussmaul respiration ('air hunger') – uncommon, has been confused with hysterical hyperventilation

May mimic acute abdomen – but acute abdomen may precipitate DKA – caution!	

Laboratory findings

Table 3.3 Laboratory findings in DKA and HHS

	DKA	HHS
Usual blood glucose (mmol/L)*	20–40	40–100+
Total fluid deficit (L)	5–8	~9
Sodium deficit (total body, mmol)	500	500
Plasma sodium[+]	Often ↓	Often high-normal or ↑
Potassium deficit (total body, mmol)	300–1000	300–1000
Plasma potassium	↓, normal or ↑	↓ or normal
Arterial pH	'Mild' DKA, 7.25–7.30 'Moderate', 7.00–7.24 'Severe', <7.0	Normal (>7.30) (unless coexisting lactic acidosis)
Arterial P_{CO_2}	↓ or normal	Normal
Base excess (mmol/L)	–10 or lower	–3 to –5
Calculated osmolality	Unreliable	>340

*Euglycamic' ketoacidosis (initial blood glucose <16.7 mmol/L) occurs in ~3% of cases; true euglycaemia (glucose <10) accounts for less than 1% of cases, but can occur when there is a prolonged vomiting illness, starvation or hyperemesis gravidarum, usually when insulin treatment has been continued. The important point is that there is no association between blood glucose level and clinical severity. Arterial pH and level of consciousness are more closely correlated.
[+]For comments on sodium levels, see text.

Ketones in DKA

The normal plasma ratio of the main ketone bodies, acetoacetate (AcAc) and β-hydroxybutyrate (β-OHB) is 1:1 (total concentration ~0.5–1.0 mmol/L). The minor ketone body acetone does not contribute to acidosis. Increased lipolysis in insulin deficiency results in excess acetyl-CoA which condenses to AcAc and is reduced to β-OHB. In untreated DKA, the β-OHB:AcAc ratio may increase to ~6:1 or more, with β-OHB concentrations up to 12 mmol/L. Once the acidosis is resolved, β-OHB is oxidised back to AcAc.

Urine ketone dipsticks detect AcAc (and acetone) but not β-OHB, so urinary ketones are an unreliable indicator of success of treatment, and they may be positive long after β-OHB has disappeared from the plasma. Simple quantitative capillary measurements of β-OHB are now available (MediSense Optium Meter [Abbott] using β-ketone electrodes) and should be used routinely in DKA, and especially when urine ketones remain positive despite a patient who is well, eating and anxious to go home. Not surprisingly, use of capillary β-OHB measurements has been shown to reduce length of stay.

ITU or PCU?

Local policies vary, but in general patients with impaired consciousness should be assessed by the ITU team, for consideration for management in a high-dependency area. These are the patients who have the most severe metabolic disturbances, and are at risk of (or may already have) cerebral oedema, which is particularly common in children and adolescents (up to 5% of cases, mortality rate up to 25%). The relatively young age and lack of comorbidity of many DKA patients should not influence decision-making; a young person in pre-coma is a high-risk patient. Other indications for intensive monitoring are:

- shock
- coexisting surgical illness
- severe coexisting medical illness, e.g. pneumonia, myocardial infarction, rhabdomyolysis.

Investigations

- Do not waste time ordering unnecessary emergency investigations.
- A biochemical flow chart is invaluable.

Obligatory

- Urinalysis for ketones (and if available quantitative capillary β-OHB): results must be written clearly in the notes. Urinalysis should be documented as the conventional semi-quantitative measurements (negative, trace, 1+–3+) and not in pseudo-quantitative form, which may be misleading.
- Plasma glucose, urea, creatinine and electrolytes.
- Blood pH and bicarbonate. Conventionally an arterial blood gas sample is used, but unless there is suspicion of hypoxia, venous blood is adequate.

- Full blood count and CRP. Ketosis itself causes neutrophilia, but there is no clear agreement on what WBC value constitutes non-specific elevation. Assess for presence of infection clinically and with CRP/ESR.
- Place a large i.v. line at the same time.

According to clinical circumstances

- ECG in patients over 40 (then maintain on a cardiac monitor – for detection of arrhythmias, and crude monitoring of potassium levels).
- Chest x-ray.
- Cultures: blood, urine, throat, CSF, septic site (always quickly check the feet for painless infected ulcers); signs of infection are likely to be blunted by acidosis.
- Creatine kinase: rhabdomyolysis is described in both DKA and HHS. Consider the possibility where there is high glucose and osmolality, and possibly low phosphate; biochemical evidence of renal failure; or clinically 'dark' urine.
- Phosphate and magnesium, where there is severe metabolic disturbance (see below).

Non-specific laboratory tests

- ↑WBC
- Abnormal liver function tests
- Amylase (allow up to 3× ULN).

Management

Fluid, potassium and insulin should be given at the same time (Table 3.4).

The main dangers are:

- circulatory collapse (hypovolaemia, acidosis, electrolyte disturbance)
- cerebral oedema – an unexpected and sudden cause of death, especially in children. The pathogenesis is not clear, but it is associated with massive fluid over-replacement and rapid changes in osmolality
- pulmonary oedema in older people, again with fluid over-replacement

Table 3.4 Management

Fluid	Potassium	Insulin
Always start with isotonic NaCl (154 mmol/L)	Add 20 mmol KCl to the first litre of NaCl if initial plasma [K+] <4 mmol/L and adequate diuresis is observed	Use continuous intravenous insulin infusion, initially at a fixed dose, e.g. 6 units/h
Treat hypotension with isotonic saline and/or plasma expanders When blood glucose <14 mmol/L, change NaCl to either 5% or 10% dextrose, and adjust insulin infusion accordingly	Thereafter, add: 40 mmol/L if [K+] <3.5 mmol/L 20 mmol/L if [K+] 3.5–5.0 mmol/L Zero if [K+] >5.0 mmol/L	

- hypokalaemia, not hyperkalaemia, especially if [K+] is low or low-normal to begin with. Severe hypokalaemia (e.g. K+ <3.3 mmol/L) – stop insulin infusion temporarily, and give 40 mmol KCl with 1 litre normal saline over 1 hour.

Fluid replacement

The aim is to replace ~6 litres within about 24 hours. An approximate regimen would be as shown in Table 3.5, but this is for guidance only; the clinical state of the patient must be carefully watched, especially for signs of fluid overload and decreasing levels of consciousness. If the patient is not particularly unwell and is not hypotensive, there is no justification for the common scenario of 1 litre saline 'stat', followed by a further 1 or 2 litres over the course of an hour or two, especially if accompanied by high-dose intravenous insulin. Hypernatraemia, failure to resolve the acidosis, and increasing mental obtundation with possible cerebral oedema are real risks. Fluid should generally be replaced more cautiously in HHS than in DKA.

Table 3.5   Fluid replacement regimen

	Duration of each litre of NaCl (h)					
DKA	1	2	2	4	4	6
HHS	2	2	4	4	8	8

Isotonic (0.9%) or 'half-normal' (0.45%) saline?

This is controversial. Isotonic saline is hypotonic (153 mmol/L) compared with the dehydrated extra- and intracellular fluid. However, hypernatraemia (serum [Na$^+$] >150 mmol/L) is a frequent problem in both DKA and HHS. Quite often this occurs because severe hyperglycaemia causes initial hyponatraemia, due to osmotic effects from water moving out of cells:

- an increase of 3.4 mmol/L in serum glucose will reduce serum [Na$^+$] by 1 mmol/L
- a serum glucose of ~40 mmol/L will therefore reduce [Na$^+$] by ~12 mmol/L.

Once rehydrated, a patient with even an initially low serum [Na$^+$] but a high initial glucose may become hypernatraemic. Consider using 0.45% saline in the presence of severe hyperglycaemia and a high-normal or high corrected [Na$^+$] after the first litre or two of isotonic saline. Note that the hypertriglyceridaemia of uncontrolled diabetes resulting from insulin deficiency does not cause hyponatraemia with modern laboratory methods for measuring electrolytes (triglycerides are not osmotically active).

Intravenous insulin regimen and blood glucose monitoring

Variable or constant rate insulin infusion?

In severe hyperglycaemia, most glucose disposal occurs through non-insulin-dependent mechanisms (e.g. renal) and this is the reason why blood glucose levels initially fall rapidly, regardless of the rate of infusion of insulin. In DKA, insulin is given primarily to suppress ketogenesis, and not to reduce blood glucose levels – which will fall in any case because of rehydration and correction of the acidosis.

In both DKA and HHS, start the insulin infusion at 6 units/h (give soluble insulin (Actrapid, Humulin S) via syringe pump – 50 mL 0.9%

29

saline with 50 units insulin). Once blood glucose levels have fallen to <14 mmol/L, replace saline with dextrose, 1 litre every 4–6 hours. Whether this should be 5% or 10% dextrose will depend on the individual, but the usual variable-rate insulin infusion regimens ('sliding scale') decrease infusion rates to 0.5–1 U/h at the lower end of the blood glucose range, and this rate of insulin infusion is not sufficient to inhibit ketogenesis, while increasing the risk of hypoglycaemia. Where possible, give a 10% dextrose infusion with a higher rate of insulin infusion.

Be especially careful with insulin infusions where there is severe hyperglycaemia and normal or high-normal [Na^+], a common situation in HHS. The risk of rapid osmotic shifts and severe hypernatraemia can be minimised initially by using low-dose insulin, e.g. 1–2 U/h, which can always be increased in the unlikely event of the blood glucose level not falling.

Capillary glucose: monitor every hour (or laboratory measurement until blood glucose is within the range of the meter, usually <33 mmol/L).

After the initial fall in blood glucose, try to keep it <10 mmol/L, but do not strive for normoglycaemia (3–7) as there is a high risk of hypoglycaemia, particularly if:

- patients are nil by mouth
- there is hepatic or renal impairment
- alcohol precipitated the emergency.

Where available, the best approach is to continue the constant-dose insulin infusion (~6 U/h), while adjusting the rate of 10% dextrose infusion to maintain blood glucose levels around 7–10 mmol/L. This is not always possible – where a variable-dose insulin regimen has to be used (for example, see Table 6.2, p. 73), ensure that meticulous measurements of urinary (or preferably blood) ketones are performed, if possible 4-hourly. 'Rebound' ketosis is not uncommon when a low-dose variable insulin infusion is stopped, particularly if there is an underlying reason for continuing insulin resistance, for example infection. If this occurs, reinstate 10% dextrose infusion together with higher-dose i.v. insulin.

Electrolytes

- Measure electrolytes, urea and creatinine at 4 and 8 hours, thereafter according to the clinical and biochemical state.
- Hypokalaemia, rather than hyperkalaemia, is often a problem,

because insulin and rising pH both drive extracellular potassium into cells (see above).

- Bicarbonate should not be given unless pH <7.0 and the patient is gravely ill. Give 700 mL of 1.2% NaHCO$_3$ solution over 45 minutes, together with 20 mmol KCl, and repeat until pH >7.0.
- Hypomagnesaemia and hypophosphataemia are common in DKA, but they are probably of importance only in those with the most severe metabolic disturbance. Low phosphate is associated with acute alcoholic intoxication, so DKA precipitated by alcohol is an important indication for measuring phosphate. Clinical manifestations of severe hypophosphataemia include respiratory failure, arrhythmias, hypotension, and generalised weakness. Consider replacement (potassium phosphate) in critically ill patients in an intensive care setting.
- Hyperchloraemic acidosis: after successful treatment of DKA, there may be a transient non-anion gap hyperchloraemic acidosis as ketones are replaced by chloride, especially when NaCl has been given in large quantities. This is an important reason for apparent failure to correct the pH in seriously ill patients.

Miscellaneous

- Unconscious patients should have urinary catheter and nasogastric tubes, but such patients should normally be managed on an ITU/PCU.
- Antibiotics should be used freely in these susceptible patients, according to the clinical situation and results of cultures, particularly in the elderly, where urinary tract and chest infections are common precipitants of HHS. Remember that patients with advanced neuropathy may be unaware of pleuritic or ischaemic chest pain or dysuria, and that ketosis suppresses fever. If there is any suspicion of infection, most clinicians would treat with, for example, co-amoxiclav, after taking appropriate cultures.
- Anticoagulation is a contentious issue, but use prophylactic anticoagulation in HHS patients, and in immobile or unconscious DKA patients.
- Keep meticulous fluid balance charts.

Follow-up

The first 12 hours of a hyperglycaemic emergency are usually managed with few problems. Thereafter, the transition to discharge can be difficult.

- Establish the cause of the emergency. The diabetes team, and in particular the diabetes specialist nurses, should be informed of all hyperglycaemic emergency admissions. An educational review is mandatory; many DKA patients are poor clinic attenders, and may already have microvascular complications. A definitive follow-up plan must be formulated and agreed with the patient; a further diabetes nurse review should be organised within a few days of discharge. A routine clinic appointment, while valuable, is unlikely to happen soon enough.
- Duration of intravenous insulin infusion. In moderate-severe DKA/HHS, most patients will require 24 hours of intravenous insulin, but if ketosis, the main problem, resolves, and there are no serious underlying problems, then patients can be transferred to subcutaneous insulin as soon as they are eating. Most patients can be discharged within 2 days. If ketonuria persists, while the patient is well and eating, confirm the absence of true ketosis by measuring capillary β-OHB (see above).
- Discontinue the i.v. regime, where possible, early in the day. If not, continue until the next day.
- Changing from i.v. to s.c. insulin: give s.c. insulin and discontinue the i.v. insulin infusion 30 minutes later, at the same time as food is given. Do not discontinue i.v. insulin before a s.c. dose has been given – food may be delayed (or not eaten) for various reasons.

Hyperosmolar patients with persistently negative ketonuria

Hyperosmolar patients with persistently negative ketonuria can often be transferred to oral hypoglycaemic agents (OHAs) before discharge:

- start patients on a sulphonylurea, e.g. gliclazide 40–80 mg b.d.
- do not use metformin, at least initially – it acts too slowly under these circumstances and there are likely to be contraindications to its use, especially impaired renal function (see Chapter 7)
- patients should be observed in hospital for at least 24 hours after transition to oral medication
- some patients will eventually be controlled on diet alone, and if this is a first presentation of diabetes, lifestyle resolve will be at its maximum at this stage – so do not use high doses of OHAs initially. Patients should be educated about hypoglycaemia – there is a wide-

spread belief that only patients on insulin can become hypogly-caemic – and ensure a follow-up appointment in the diabetes clinic or with the patient's own practice clinic is made within a week or two.

Known type 1 patients

The previous insulin regimen should be re-established unless it is clearly responsible for the episode of DKA (very unusual). It is pointless making substantive changes while an in-patient; any changes can be much better made in the out-patient setting.

Newly diagnosed type 1 patients

Most in time will do best with a multiple-dose (basal-bolus) regimen, but there is controversy about whether this should be the discharge regimen in a newly diagnosed patient. It will largely depend on the support available – if it is intensive, then it might be practicable, but the most important considerations early on are:

- avoiding hypoglycaemia
- suppressing ketogenesis

and these require relatively small doses of insulin. In routine practice, it is often best to use a twice-daily premixed soluble or soluble analogue/isophane mixture, preferably given with a pen device. Start with either Mixtard 30 or Humulin M3, given 30 minutes before breakfast and evening meal, or NovoMix 30 or Humalog Mix 25 given with meals.

Patients may be in 'honeymoon', with partial and temporary recovery of β-cell function, so they should be started with small doses, e.g. 10–12 units with/before breakfast, 6–8 units with/before evening meal, perhaps even less in underweight or small patients. The widely used rule of taking the previous 24-hour intravenous insulin infusion requirements, and dividing by 2 or 4, is not physiologically sound, and is likely to result in hypoglycaemia, especially when the patient becomes more physically active after discharge.

However, do not be too relaxed about glycaemic control in the early stages of type 1 diabetes. The Diabetes Control and Complications Trial (DCCT) found that about one-third of type 1 patients with duration <5 years have some residual insulin secretion, and that intensive treatment of these patients, i.e. HbA$_{1c}$ ≤7.0%, can help sustain endogenous insulin secretion – with benefits for metabolic control and lower risks of hypoglycaemia and microvascular complications.

Hypoglycaemia

Every patient presenting to an A&E department with impaired consciousness must have a reliable blood glucose measurement performed on admission, and the result formally recorded. Hypoglycaemia is the commonest complication of type 1 diabetes, and is frequent in type 2 patients treated with insulin or with sulphonylureas. An attempt should always be made to determine the cause of the hypoglycaemia; it will determine future management, and may be life-saving.

Causes

Singly, or in combination, these factors account for the majority of episodes of hypoglycaemia:

- dietary: missing or delaying a meal
- too much insulin: inadvertent administration
- unaccustomed exercise
- alcohol.

However, more uncommon causes should also be considered:

- overdosage of insulin or sulphonylureas: unexpected factitious sulphonylurea overdosage in patients with documented severe hypoglycaemia is surprisingly common. Sulphonylureas can be measured in urine and plasma. Factitious insulin overdosage can be diagnosed by detecting high insulin and low C-peptide levels. Insulin-sensitising agents (metformin and glitazones) do not cause significant hypoglycaemia
- newly developed endocrine disease, especially Addison's disease (increased risk in patients with type 1 diabetes) and hypopituitarism. Onset may be insidious – Addison's disease should always be considered in a type 1 patient whose insulin dose falls by more than ~20% as a response to frequent hypoglycaemia
- impaired absorption: gastroenteritis, coeliac disease
- impaired gastric emptying: gastroparesis (autonomic neuropathy)
- failure to decrease insulin dose post-partum; breast feeding

- early pregnancy (decreased insulin requirements and nausea/hyper-mesis).

Remember also the non-diabetic causes of hypoglycaemia – insulinoma, hypothermia, alcohol and drugs:

- Severe hypoglycaemia has been reported in patients taking glibenclamide who are prescribed fluoroquinolone antibiotics (glibenclamide is metabolised by the P-450 hepatic system; fluoroquinolones inhibit the same system).
- Non-steroidal anti-inflammatory drugs (including aspirin) can also potentiate the actions of sulphonylureas.
- Combinations of drugs might contribute to hypoglycaemia in patients already in good glycaemic control, e.g. β-blockers, ACE inhibitors.

Operational classification of hypoglycaemia

Biochemical/asymptomatic
Biochemical counterregulation in the non-diabetic person starts when blood glucose levels fall to <3.8 mmol/L. This is very common, especially at night in type 1 patients. Multiple studies confirm that motor responses are impaired at this level, particularly important when driving. Many patients believe that hypoglycaemia means only impaired consciousness. Correcting this misconception is an important educational point; 'four's the floor' (i.e. avoid blood glucose levels <4 mmol/L) is a useful mnemonic.

Treatment
When asymptomatic blood glucose levels <4.0 mmol/L are detected, patients should take or be offered prophylactic treatment. This is especially important if patients are taking intermediate- or long-acting insulin, or are likely to miss their next meal. It should go without saying that appropriate dose reductions in insulin or OHAs should be made if biochemical hypoglycaemia is frequent; but unfortunately it still needs saying.

Mild (self-treated) symptomatic hypoglycaemia
Most well-controlled type 1 patients experience about two mild hypoglycaemic episodes each week. Symptoms are variable, but in individuals they are often stereotyped in nature and sequence:

- autonomic: sweating, hunger, trembling, anxiety, pounding heart
- neuroglycopenic: confusion, odd behaviour, difficulty concentrating
- motor: incoordination, difficulty walking
- sensory: visual disturbance, perioral tingling
- others: headache, nausea, difficulty speaking.

Treatment
Patients should take at least 20 g carbohydrate. This is contained in, for example:

- two slices of bread
- a snack-size chocolate bar
- 100 mL Lucozade
- 300 mL non-diet cola drink
- three cubes of sugar (sucrose).

There is little difference between these in absorption characteristics, though liquid is usually recommended. A glycaemic response occurs in 10–15 minutes, though the symptomatic response is usually more rapid. There is no point in repeating blood glucose measurements after a shorter interval.

Severe hypoglycaemia
Severe hypoglycaemia is defined as an event in which the patient needs the assistance of another person.

- ~10% of type 1 patients have an episode of severe hypoglycaemia each year, rising to ~30% in intensively treated patients. ~3% of insulin-treated type 2 patients have a similar episode each year.
- ~3% have recurrent severe hypoglycaemia. Even in this group, there is surprisingly little evidence for long-term intellectual impairment.
- The rates in patients treated with OHAs are much lower, ~0.5% per year.

Most patients are aware of autonomic symptoms at glucose levels of 2–3 mmol/L (experimental threshold is ~3.2 mmol/L) but patients with habitual low glucose levels will have a degree of hypoglycaemia unawareness, and may be apparently fully alert and responsive at levels of ~1–2 mmol/L, though impairment of cognitive function invariably occurs below 3 mmol/L. Family members, friends and co-workers are frequently more sensitive at detecting subtle behavioural signs of hypoglycaemia than the patient.

Risk factors for severe hypoglycaemia

- Intensive insulin therapy (multiple daily doses of insulin or CSII).
- Low HbA_{1c} levels, often in the non-diabetic range, e.g. 4–6%.
- Sleep and alcohol: alcohol induces early hyperglycaemia, but late hypoglycaemia, which may occur at the same time as the maximum effect of a late-night dose of isophane insulin (this is itself a good reason for suggesting a change to a long-acting analogue in young people particularly at risk of alcohol-induced hypoglycaemia).
- Hypoglycaemia unawareness: risk factors are increasing duration of insulin treatment; age (elderly and the very young); previous hypoglycaemic episodes; established autonomic neuropathy is not consistently a factor, though autonomic neuropathy is associated with long-duration diabetes.
- Pancreatic diabetes, usually associated with alcoholism, due to absent glucagon secretion, through destruction of α cells.
- Social isolation.

Strict avoidance of hypoglycaemia for about 3 weeks can restore hypoglycaemia awareness, but this requires intensive management with frequent home blood glucose testing.

The unusual presentations of severe hypoglycaemia are:

- seizure
- hemiparesis
- aggressive (possibly criminal) behaviour
- 'He's been drinking, doctor'
- acute back pain – opisthotonos or rarely crush fracture of thoracic vertebra caused by fits.

Treatment

Intravenous glucose: 20–30 ml of 50% dextrose (10–15 g glucose) given by bolus intravenous injection into a large peripheral vein. Potential problems are:

- viscous solution: may be difficult to inject, particularly in a restless patient
- occasional phlebitis (with both intra- and extravascular placement)
- gaining venous access in patients who have often had repeated previous infusions. Wherever possible, try to avoid using the peripheral veins of the legs.

Glucagon, a major insulin antagonist hormone, is useful in management by paramedics out of hospital, and as an initial treatment in the unconscious or restless patient where venous access is delayed. It is presented as a standard preparation of 1 mg. It acts through direct stimulation of hepatic glycogenolysis, and is therefore:

- relatively ineffective in the patient with poor hepatic glycogen stores – thin, malnourished, starving, anorectic or alcoholic
- relatively effective in the patient with predominant glucagon deficiency, e.g. pancreatic diabetes
- usually clinically effective in 20 minutes
- usually transient in its effect (~90 minutes) and must be supplemented by oral glucose as soon as the patient is capable of taking it.

It can be given i.v., i.m., or s.c., but i.m. is preferable because the s.c. route may not be so effective in vasoconstricted patients, and i.v. injection may cause nausea.

Glucagon stimulates insulin release, so should not be used in hypoglycaemia caused by sulphonylureas.

Follow-up
- After initial treatment in A&E, replenish hepatic glycogen stores by giving a substantial carbohydrate-containing snack after recovery – 3–6 biscuits, bread or sandwiches – to prevent recurrent hypoglycaemia.
- Check a further capillary blood glucose level after 20 minutes.
- If patients have recovered, are fully conscious and have a blood glucose level >7 mmol/L within 1 hour, admission is not required, but arrangements must be made for prompt follow-up by the diabetes team, especially if there is no obvious reason for the episode.

When to admit

- Patients with residual neurological deficits or prolonged coma after treatment – postictal state, cerebral oedema, head injury, intracranial infection, bleed or infarction, and coexisting poisoning with alcohol or drugs should be considered. Get an urgent brain CT scan.
- Patients who live on their own with no facilities for close monitoring over the next 24 hours.

- Sulphonylurea-induced hypoglycaemia, which may require prolonged treatment with 10 or 20% dextrose.
- Recurrent hypoglycaemia, despite adequate treatment. This suggests:
  - liver disease
  - massive insulin overdose, intentional or otherwise
  - long-acting sulphonylurea.

4 ACUTE GENERAL MEDICINE AND DIABETES

Rigorous control of blood glucose levels is required in:

- acute coronary syndromes
- intensive care
- perioperative care (see Chapter 6).

Other common clinical situations are:

- blood glucose control in non-critically ill patients
- stroke
- capillary blood glucose monitoring
- enteral feeding
- glucocorticoid treatment
- in-patient screening routine.

Acute coronary syndromes (ACS)

Once infarction has occurred, all outcomes are worse in diabetic, compared with non-diabetic subjects with mortality rates consistently 50–60% higher; early excess mortality is particularly pronounced, but continues, at least in historical studies, up to 5 years. Several factors are involved.

- Classical (textbook) ischaemic symptoms are less marked or absent, presumably due to somatic and autonomic neuropathy (think of ischaemia in a diabetic patient who describes shortness of breath, nausea/vomiting, sweating, even non-specific upper body discomfort). Patients are unlikely to describe classical symptoms if English is not their first language.
- Hospital presentation is later, and thrombolysis and percutaneous coronary intervention may be delayed.
- Coronary artery disease is more diffuse and more advanced, and associated risk factors more marked.

The extent of infarction is probably no greater than in non-diabetic subjects, but disease in other coronary artery territories may account for the increased complication rate. However, results from DIGAMI 2 (see below) suggest that with the most vigorous modern treatments, long-term outcomes need not be dissimilar from those in non-diabetic patients.

Many patients with myocardial infarction (MI) and no prior history of diabetes have abnormal glucose tolerance; the prevalence rates are similar immediately after the event and some months later:

- 50% normal glucose tolerance
- 30% impaired glucose tolerance
- 20% diabetes.

There is therefore a powerful case for attempting a formal diagnosis of the glucose tolerance status of all ACS patients. There are no guidelines; because of the abnormal acute metabolic state, even diagnostic levels (random glucose levels ≥ 11.1 mmol/L) should be formally confirmed, but random admission glucose measurements of ≥ 7.0 mmol/L or $HbA_{1c} > 6.0$–6.5% should be regarded as suspicious. This is one situation in which routine admission HbA_{1c} measurements might be justified.

Glycaemic control

Use of glucose-insulin-potassium (GIK) infusions in the acute phase of MI has a long history; the metabolic reasoning includes conversion of the less efficient myocardial metabolism of free fatty acids to the more efficient glucose metabolism.

The first DIGAMI study (1997) showed that treatment of MI patients who had an admission blood glucose >11.1 mmol/L (nearly all of whom had true diabetes, either known or newly diagnosed) with intravenous GIK for at least 24 hours, followed by 3 months of basal-bolus subcutaneous insulin, decreased the absolute risk of fatal reinfarction over the next 3.5 years by 11%, but had no effect on total reinfarctions. Benefit was similar in patients with previously diagnosed and newly presenting diabetes, and was particularly notable in patients at low risk (e.g. under 70 years, no previous infarct or heart failure, and not treated with digoxin).

DIGAMI 2 (2004) attempted to determine the importance of the acute and long-term phase of tight blood glucose control in improving prognosis. The study failed; it was stopped early because of inadequate recruitment, and was statistically underpowered and, not surprisingly, there were no differences between the three groups studied: (1) GIK for

24 hours, followed by s.c. insulin; (2) GIK for 24 hours, followed by 'conventional' treatment; and (3) conventional treatment only. Mean admission HbA$_{1c}$ was already very good (7.3%), so significant improvement was difficult to achieve, and there was less than 1 mmol/L difference in blood glucose levels between the groups. The cardiac outcomes were the same as, possibly even better than, those in a concurrent registry cohort, and the investigators concluded that with vigorous management of all factors (of which tight glycaemic control is one, but only one; for example 40% of patients had primary revascularisation), outcomes could be markedly improved in this high-risk group.

In practice, giving insulin for 24 hours in the acute phase is simple, and all hyperglycaemic patients (admission blood glucose >11 mmol/L) should probably continue to have this treatment, though see below for a more recent large-scale study. The acute DIGAMI regimen is complex, so most units use a variable dose insulin infusion together with 5% dextrose, aiming for capillary blood glucose (CBG) levels of 7–10 mmol/L. Whether this confers the same benefit is not known. DIGAMI 2 suggests that s.c. insulin following this is less important than achieving good overall glycaemic control (targets – not met – were fasting 5–7 mmol/L, post-prandial 7–10) using any means. A certain proportion of patients will benefit from insulin (see Chapter 7) but many will achieve these levels with intensification of the OHA regimen, and strict attention to diet and exercise. Because of their actual (metformin) or likely (glitazone) cardiac benefits, these agents should be employed wherever possible. Metformin, unless contraindicated for other reasons, should always be reinstated after coronary interventions.

The huge CREATE-ECLA study (2005) randomised ~20 000 STEMI patients, of whom ~3500 had type 2 diabetes, to usual care or usual care + high dose GIK for 24 hours (25% glucose, 50 U/L soluble insulin, 80 mmol/L KCl infused at 1.5 mL/kg/h). There was no benefit either on mortality or serious cardiovascular end points at 30 days, in the whole group or in the diabetic subjects. Although blood glucose levels were relatively poorly controlled (8–10 mmol/L), this substantial study casts some doubt on the utility of this widely-used and historically long-used treatment.

Thrombolysis

With the introduction of care pathways, diabetic patients currently are as likely to receive thrombolysis as non-diabetic patients, a significant change over the past 10 years – though there are likely to be local variations. Thrombolysis achieves as good epicardial blood flow in diabetic as in non-diabetic subjects, and bleeding complications are similar, but complete ST segment resolution is less frequent. However, in long-term follow-up, absolute benefit remains greater in diabetes.

Contraindications are similar to those in non-diabetic subjects. Retinopathy of any degree, even laser treated, is not a contraindication, and fundoscopy is unnecessary and wastes time.

Primary percutaneous coronary intervention (PCI)

This is a rapidly changing and specialist field. However, in general, outcomes are worse in diabetic, compared with non-diabetic, patients. Preprocedural clopidogrel, followed by 1 year of maintenance treatment, decreases long-term clinical events.

ST-segment elevation myocardial infarction (STEMI)

Where available, angioplasty with stenting and platelet glycoprotein (GP) IIb/IIIa inhibitor treatment improves outcomes in diabetic and non-diabetic patients compared with fibrinolytic therapy.

Non-ST-segment elevation myocardial infarction (NSTEMI) and NSTE acute coronary syndromes

Management is controversial. Patients with diabetes appear to be the only group benefiting from GP IIb/IIIa inhibitor therapy, a benefit that is even greater if PCI is performed during the index hospitalisation. Unfortunately, these options are not usually available in the UK at present. In general, diabetic patients benefit more from a deliberate strategy of intensive medical management, followed by early angiography and revascularisation.

Coronary angioplasty (PTCA), stents and coronary artery bypass (CABG)

Single-vessel intervention

Angioplasty has been supplanted by stenting, and the DIABETES study (2005) showed that diabetic, like non-diabetic patients, had better outcomes (0% stent thrombosis, lower rate of revascularisation and major cardiac events) when sirolimus-coated stents are used instead of the older bare metal stents, in predominantly multivessel interventions. The SIRIUS study (2003–04) gave similar results in single-vessel disease,

44

although diabetic patients still had a higher frequency of repeat intervention, especially if they were insulin-treated, though this is not likely to be a causative association. Sirolimus-eluting stents appear to carry a lower risk of in-stent restenosis in both diabetic and non-diabetic patients than paclitaxel-eluting stents (ISAR-DIABETES, 2005).

Multivessel disease

The first BARI study (1996) found that CABG carried a better 5-year survival rate in diabetic (though not in non-diabetic) patients. However, this study was carried out in the pre-stent era, and there is optimism, though no clear evidence as yet, that diabetic patients may benefit as much from multiple drug-eluting stents as from CABG. BARI 2D (PCI versus intensive medical management; insulin-replacing versus insulin-sensitising treatment, target HbA_{1c} <7.0%) will not complete for several years.

Intensive care

Hyperglycaemia in critically ill patients (with or without diabetes) carries a poor prognosis (vascular disease, polyneuropathy, increased tendency to infection, dyslipidaemia, and abnormal anti-inflammatory and coagulation responses) – just as in established diabetes. Rigorous blood glucose control if blood glucose >6.1 mmol/L (target blood glucose 4.5–6.0 mmol/L) compared with conventional control (insulin therapy only if blood glucose >12 mmol/L, target 10–11 mmol/L) markedly improved outcomes in all patients who needed >5 days ICU treatment: intensive care and hospital survival, duration of ventilatory support, length of ICU stay, septic complications, critical illness polyneuropathy and acute renal failure. Although this was in a ventilated group of predominantly surgical and trauma patients, this simple and remarkably effective treatment (mechanism not yet clear) can now be generalised to other ICU patients. Most intensive care settings have specific protocols for ensuring near-normoglycaemia in these cases. The cardiac and ITU studies imply that a combination of intensive/high dose insulin therapy and near-normoglycaemia are required for optimum outcomes.

Blood glucose control in non-critically ill patients

There is no evidence that intensive blood glucose control in patients not in the above groups improves prognosis, but every attempt should be made to avoid hypoglycaemia and blood glucose levels consistently >12–15 mmol/L. This is often difficult to achieve with OHA or twice-daily fixed mixture s.c. insulin treatment, but if the patient is eating, a temporary change to a basal-bolus insulin regimen, with frequent changes in doses on the basis of CBG monitoring, will usually be satisfactory. However, there is no point in changing a regimen if the admission is likely to be short.

If the patient is not eating, then use a continuous variable insulin infusion together with 5% or 10% dextrose. However, this should not be continued for long periods because of the discomfort, inconvenience, and risk of electrolyte disturbances (especially hyponatraemia).

Stroke

In many clinical studies the degree of hyperglycaemia at presentation has been found to be related to:

- initial infarct volume
- early infarct progression
- poor early and medium-term clinical outcomes.

Stroke patients have a high prevalence of hyperglycaemia, and newly diagnosed diabetes is common in stroke survivors, with a similar rate to that in MI (40% of survivors have normal glucose tolerance, 40% IGT, 20% diabetes). Admission plasma glucose ≥6.1 mmol/L together with HbA_{1c} ≥6.2% is predictive of diabetes at follow-up.

Studies are in progress to determine the benefits of acute control of hyperglycaemia (targeting levels 4–7 mmol/L), but there is no definitive evidence as yet. Current European guidelines advocate glucose levels <10 mmol/L, American guidelines <16.6 mmol/L.

In practice, hypoglycaemia poses a more serious risk to the stroke patient than moderate hyperglycaemia. In a stroke unit or emergency admission unit, it would be reasonable to use the same protocol as MI patients, i.e. 24 hours of a variable insulin infusion + 5% dextrose, or GIK infusion, with hourly blood glucose monitoring, in patients with admission glucose >10 mmol/L (<20% of patients). However, unless close monitoring can be guaranteed, this should not be used in patients who are comatose or who have severely impaired consciousness. Even without insulin treatment, glucose levels tend to fall over the first 8 hours after admission in stroke patients, so do not rush to start an intravenous regimen.

Capillary blood glucose monitoring

Blood glucose monitoring is uncomfortable for patients, and time-consuming. It must be used appropriately and the testing sticks and meters in use in hospital should be familiar to doctors so that, if necessary, they can make a reliable measurement. Indicate on the appropriate monitoring sheet and communicate to the nurses:

- times for blood glucose monitoring
- when times should be reviewed.

Pre-meal monitoring takes place immediately before meals; post-meal monitoring, 90 minutes after meals. Only unstable or perioperative patients require 7-point blood glucose series (pre- and post-meal, and pre-bedtime); otherwise monitoring is done according to circumstances:

- patients on twice-daily fixed mixture: pre- and post lunch and pre-bed
- patients on basal-bolus regimen: fasting, one or two other measurements during the day.

CBG <4.0 should be treated as hypoglycaemia, regardless of the patient's symptoms (see Chapter 3). Subsequently, blood glucose testing should focus around the time(s) of hypoglycaemia and appropriate reductions in insulin doses or OHA made if there is a consistent pattern. Although patients often have insulin-resistant conditions while in hospital, they are also often eating less than usual.

Enteral feeding (nasogastric, PEG)

This frequently results in severe hyperglycaemia, often requiring insulin. The clinical problem is usually the very rapid rise in glucose levels after the start of the feed. Try a fixed mixture with a rapid acting analogue at the start of the feed, e.g. Humalog Mix 50, starting at 16–20 units; isophane or long-acting analogue has little chance of picking up the initial blood glucose surge. A once-daily regimen may be suitable, particularly if there is a 12–14 hour feed period, followed by water. If there is continuous feeding, try either a twice-daily mixture, or two injections at the start of the feed, e.g. Actrapid/Humulin S 8-10 units + Lantus/Levemir ~20 units. Discuss the feeding regime with the dietician and the nursing staff.

Glucocorticoid treatment

Acute, high-dosage corticosteroid treatment, e.g. prednisolone >20–30 mg daily, 'neurological' doses of dexamethasone (e.g. 16 mg/day), nearly always causes marked deterioration in glycaemic control in known diabetic patients, especially post-prandially. The mechanism is increased peripheral insulin resistance, but this fact is of little practical help, because severe acute hyperglycaemia is unlikely to respond to drugs that would rationally reduce insulin resistance, e.g. metformin, glitazones. Sulphonylureas and insulin are the mainstays of treatment.

There are no clear guidelines for the management of acute steroid-induced diabetes, and it is not clear in what proportion of patients it remits once treatment is stopped. Clinically, remission is more likely in those who do not have pretreatment evidence of insulin resistance (thin, non-hypertensive).

The aim in short-term steroid treatment is to relieve symptoms; the usual criteria for good control would apply in long-term treatment.

Management

Patients with known diabetes

Insulin-treated diabetes

Increased insulin requirements of 25–50% should be anticipated, so start increasing insulin doses as soon as steroid treatment starts.

OHA-treated diabetes

- Increase the dose of sulphonylurea according to blood glucose measurements. Remember, if patients are already taking near-maximum doses (e.g. glibenclamide 10–15 mg/day, gliclazide 160–240 mg/day, glimepiride 2–3 mg/day), they are very likely to need insulin treatment.
- Continue metformin and glitazones in pre-existing doses, unless contraindicated, but do not increase the doses in an attempt to control rising blood glucose levels – they act too slowly to be effective in this situation. Do not withdraw sulphonylureas, but watch for hypoglycaemia.
- Convert to insulin sooner rather than later, certainly when random

CBG >15, at which levels hyperglycaemic symptoms are likely to occur.

- Start with twice-daily fixed mixtures, e.g. Mixtard 30, NovoMix 30, Humulin M3, Humalog Mix 25, e.g. 12 units a.m., 8 units p.m., and be prepared to increase each dose daily by at least 2 units. Basal-bolus regimens may be useful in long-term treatment.

Non-diabetic patients

Monitoring
Daily urinalysis, and random CBG preferentially 2 hours after meals:

- CBG up to 10 → diet
- CBG 10–15 → sulphonylurea
- CBG >15 → insulin.

Patients should be taught blood glucose monitoring. If the steroid dose tapers or stops abruptly, intensify monitoring. Always measure HbA_{1c} – some of these patients will have pre-existing undiagnosed diabetes.

In-patient screening routine

All diabetic patients admitted to hospital should be screened in a standard way – but this must be done sensibly, and is unnecessary until the acute phase of any illness is settled. This routine is particularly important in patients:

- admitted with a hyperglycaemic emergency, especially type 1 patients with DKA
- who have little or no contact with their primary care teams, and may not have been screened for complications.

Clinical examination

- Peripheral vascular disease
- Arterial bruits
- Feet
- Weight and body mass index.

Dilated fundoscopy

Unless there is evidence of a formal eye review within the past year, the pupils should be dilated, the fundi examined, and the findings recorded in the notes. If there is retinopathy that is likely to need laser treatment (see Chapter 9), the patient should be referred directly to the eye team.

Blood tests

Diabetic patients with general medical or surgical illnesses have countless blood counts and renal and liver function tests, but blood should also be taken for:

- HbA_{1c}
- fasting lipids
- thyroid function tests (if not tested within the past 5 years).

Other tests

- Urinalysis, especially for ketones and protein.
- 24-hour urinary albumin measurement. Although elevated by infection, fever or severe hyperglycaemia, it will give a good indication of the likely range of albuminuria out of acute illness.
- 12 lead ECG.
- Dietetic review, as required.
- Review with diabetes specialist nurses for insulin-taking patients – if possible identify in advance likely areas that will need addressing:
    - insulin regimen – did it directly or indirectly cause the admission? Can it be rationalised and/or simplified? Is the patient using up-to-date equipment?
    - injection technique
    - home blood glucose monitoring and equipment
    - employment, school, driving status, family psychodynamics, alcohol, smoking and drugs.

5 INSULIN THERAPY IN TYPE 1 DIABETES

Figures 5.1, 5.2 and 5.3 show results of continuous glucose monitoring studies using a subcutaneous sensor (MiniMed) to record interstitial glucose levels in real time over a prolonged period (up to 5 days). Patients do normal activities on their usual insulin regimens out of hospital throughout this time. The glucose levels are not accessible at the time of recording. Each line represents one day of recording. In these pictures they are superimposed.

Insulin treatment in type 1 diabetes is substitution/replacement therapy, but replacement is much more variable and difficult than in other hormone deficiencies (e.g. thyroid, adrenal) because of the minute-to-minute control of blood glucose levels exerted by the intact pancreas, which cannot be emulated precisely by any current subcutaneous insulin regimen. You are unlikely ever to encounter two type 1 patients (or even type 2 patients) taking identical insulin regimens, and there is usually room for improving control in type 1 diabetes using different insulin regimens.

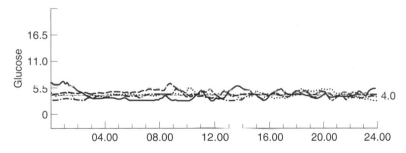

Figure 5.1 Non-diabetic subject (investigated for possible hypoglycaemia). The astonishing consistency and narrowness of the range of normal glucose levels is apparent, with transient slight increases noticeable after breakfast and lunch – but values are never higher than ~7 mmol/L. Usual levels are 3–4 mmol/L. (Continuous glucose monitoring is a valuable technique for the preliminary investigation of non-diabetic hypoglycaemia; in this case the patient had no significant symptoms, and no glucose levels <3 mmol/L).

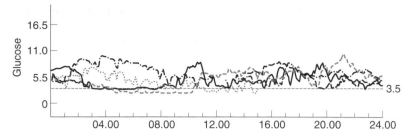

Figure 5.2 Continuous glucose monitoring study in a 27-year-old type 1 patient, duration 15 years. This is good control (HbA$_{1c}$ 7%) in a patient using up to five injections of insulin a day, but note the wider range of glucose values (frequently 8–10), together with 4–7 hours of significant hypoglycaemia (glucose ≤3.5 mmol/L) on two nights. There are brief periods of hypoglycaemia during the day.

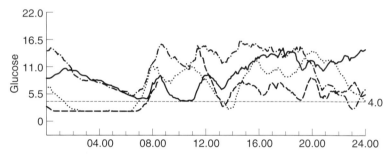

Figure 5.3 More typical glucose levels in a 40-year-old type 1 patient, duration 17 years, average HbA$_{1c}$ 8.5%. Basal-bolus regimen, 10–14 units soluble insulin with meals, long-acting analogue (glargine) 14 units at night. Note the wide excursions, with long-lasting overnight hypoglycaemia on two out of four nights (long-acting analogues reduce the risk of nocturnal hypoglycaemia, but do not reliably abolish it), and the marked post-prandial peaks, especially after breakfast and lunch. He has no detectable microvascular complications.

Insulin is an anabolic hormone, and there is increasing concern, mostly from the DCCT results, but from other prospective studies in type 1 diabetes as well, of the following process: poor glycaemic control → intensive glycaemic control → increased weight → increasing

52

insulin resistance → increased risks of macrovascular disease and microvascular disease, especially nephropathy.

There is therefore a difficult balance to achieve between:

- overinsulinisation and weight gain with increasing insulin resistance, and increased risks of hypoglycaemia, but perhaps improved HbA_{1c}
- reducing frequency of severe hypoglycaemia (which also causes weight increase)
- avoiding persistent severe hyperglycaemia with the attendant long-term risks of microvascular complications.

Glycaemic targets in type 1 diabetes

The question of a glycaemic 'threshold' for the development of microvascular complications has not been resolved.

HbA_{1c} <7.5% is a widely accepted and realistic figure (ADA proposes <7.0% for all adults with diabetes). Further protection could be expected with lower values, but at the expense of increased risk of hypoglycaemia. This risk is particularly high with HbA_{1c} levels consistently <~6.0–6.5%.

Targets for capillary glucose values are:

- pre-prandial: 5.0–7.2 mmol/L
- post-prandial: <10.0 mmol/L.

Relationship between HbA_{1c} and mean glucose levels

DCCT found a strong correlation between mean diurnal capillary blood glucose measurements and HbA_{1c}, the strongest association being with post-lunch blood glucose measurements. (This finding justifies measuring random CBG in patients attending afternoon diabetes clinics.) Because of the clinical relevance of mean blood glucose measurements, it is likely that HbA_{1c} measurements will soon be quoted together with their associated mean blood glucose value (Table 5.1).

Continuous glucose monitoring studies (CGMS)

Where available, continuous glucose monitoring studies (CGMS) are invaluable, as they can identify periods of the day and night where hypoglycaemia and hyperglycaemia are consistently occurring. This important technique has confirmed the following:

Table 5.1 HbA$_{1c}$ and mean capillary blood glucose values

HbA$_{1c}$ (%)	Approximate mean capillary blood glucose for clinical use (mmol/L)
5	5.0
6	6.8
7	8.5
8	10.4
9	12.1
10	14.0
11	15.8
12	17.5

- Stable blood glucose levels are almost never attainable in insulin-treated patients.
- Using conventional isophane (NPH) insulin at bedtime, many patients are frequently hypoglycaemic for long periods overnight, without waking up, and without symptoms the next day.
- Prolonged asymptomatic hypoglycaemia is frequent during the day as well.
- Post-prandial rises in blood glucose levels can be very rapid (Figure 5.3).
- Post-hypoglycaemic peaks in blood glucose (with or without glucose taken by the patient) can be very high (Figure 5.3).
- Corrective action taken on the basis of the results can significantly improve glycaemic control.
- Patterns of glycaemia are much easier to detect than with even frequent home blood glucose monitoring (HBGM); where there are rapid rises and falls in blood glucose levels, small differences in timing of insulin injections and capillary glucose measurements can give the impression of greater variability than there actually is.

Insulin preparations

Many insulin preparations are available, but most clinics become familiar with about 6–10 preparations. Manufacturers continue to rationalise their insulin ranges, and within the next few years it is likely that fewer than a dozen preparations will be in widespread use. This will help the occasional prescriber, who is as bemused by the number of insulin preparations as, for example, is the diabetologist by the variety of inhalers in use in chest medicine.

Analogue (modified human) insulins

Over the past 8 years, manufacturers have modified the human insulin molecule to alter its physicochemical characteristics in various ingenious ways to provide more precisely targeted release characteristics. The first to be introduced were the fast-acting analogues lispro and aspart, which, through a lesser tendency to aggregate into hexamers, have a more rapid onset and offset of action compared with standard soluble insulin. More recently, the long-acting analogues glargine and detemir have been devised, which provide more consistent insulin levels, resulting in more stable glucose levels for prolonged periods, especially overnight, together with a lower risk of hypoglycaemia, compared with isophane (NPH) insulin. Where they are available, all type 1 patients should have the opportunity to try these newer preparations.

Prescribing

- Precision is vital, especially when writing numbers. Errors can be fatal.
- Generic insulin is not available in the UK, so it must be prescribed by trade name.
- 'Units' should be written in full, or just the number. Do not abbreviate to 'u', which can be misread as '0', or 'iu' (international units), which can be misread as '10'.
- In-patient prescribing: the precise time of administration in relation to meals should be written, not just as clock time. Premixed insulins must not be prescribed in the middle of the day or at bedtime, an alarmingly common practice. Name any injection device in the prescription.

Formulations

- Nearly all insulin is now biosynthetic human, with only very few patients using beef or highly purified (monocomponent) pork insulins.
- All insulin in Europe and the USA is U100 (100 units/mL).
- Bottles of insulin contain 10 mL (1000 units), and cartridges 3 mL (300 units).

Most patients in the UK use insulin pens and 3 mL cartridges of insulin, rather than syringes and 10 mL bottles. Pens frequently change, but are basically of two types as follows.

Table 5.2 Insulin preparations in the UK (August 2005)

Preparation	Manufacturer	Formulations	Approximate time course of action/notes		
			Onset	Peak	Duration
Rapid-acting insulin analogues (approved name)					
Humalog (lispro)	Lilly	Vial, cartridges, Humalog pen (prefilled)	15–30 min	1 h	5 h
NovoRapid (aspart)	NovoNordisk	Vial, cartridges, Flexpen (prefilled)			
Apidra (glulisine)	Sanofi-Aventis	Vial, cartridges			
Short-acting insulin (soluble/neutral)					
Humulin S	Lilly	Vial, cartridges	30 min	1–2 h	6–8 h
Actrapid	NovoNordisk	Vial			
Insuman Rapid	Sanofi-Aventis	Cartridges, Optiset pen (prefilled)			
Intermediate-acting insulin (NPH, isophane)					
Humulin I	Lilly	Vial, cartridges, Humulin I pen (prefilled)	2 h	4–6 h	8–12 h
Insulatard	NovoNordisk	Vial, cartridges, Innolet (prefilled)			
Insuman Basal	Sanofi-Aventis	Vial, cartridges, Optiset pen (prefilled)			

Biphasic insulin ('fixed mixtures')

Name	Manufacturer	Presentation	Onset	Peak	Duration	Comment
Humulin M3 (30% soluble, 70% NPH)	Lilly	Vial, cartridges, Humulin M3 pen (prefilled)	30 min	2–6 h	8–12 h	Mixtures containing different percentages of soluble insulin, the amount denoted by the figures. Differing intensity of early action; relatively infrequently used
Mixtard 30 (30/70)	NovoNordisk	Vial, cartridges, Innolet (prefilled)				
Mixtard 10,20,40,50	NovoNordisk	Cartridges only				
Insuman Comb 25	Sanofi-Aventis	Cartridges, Optiset pen (prefilled)				
Insuman Comb 50	Sanofi-Aventis	Cartridges, Optiset pen (prefilled)				

Biphasic insulin containing rapid-acting analogues

Name	Manufacturer	Presentation	Comment
Humalog Mix 25	Lilly	Cartridges, Humalog Mix 25 pen (prefilled)	Mixtures containing different percentages of rapid-acting analogue, the amount denoted by the figures. Differing intensity of early action
Humalog Mix 50	Lilly	Humalog Mix 50 pen (prefilled)	
NovoMix 30	NovoNordisk	Cartridges, Flexpen (prefilled)	

Long-acting analogues

Name	Manufacturer	Presentation	Comment
Lantus (glargine)	Sanofi-Aventis	Vial, cartridges, Optiset pen (prefilled)	Smooth, peakless action, duration of 16-24 h
Levemir (detemir)	NovoNordisk	Cartridges, Flexpen (prefilled)	

Vial, 10 mL bottle, for use with insulin syringe; Cartridge, 3 mL cartridge for use with refillable pen; Pen, prefilled disposable pen containing 3mL cartridge.

Refillable

- NovoNordisk: NovoPen 3, NovoPen Junior (delivers in 0.5 unit increments – useful for children and adults with low insulin requirements)
- Lilly: HumaPen Luxura; HumaPen Ergo
- Sanofi-Aventis: Optipen
- Owen Mumford: Autopen 24 (Sanofi-Aventis cartridges). Other Autopens (Lilly and CP cartridges).

Prefilled, disposable pens

These are increasingly used because of convenience, safety and simplicity to teach. They are prescribed by writing the insulin type followed by the name of the pen:

- NovoNordisk: FlexPen, e.g. NovoRapid FlexPen
- Lilly: e.g. Humalog Mix25 Pen
- Sanofi-Aventis: Optiset, e.g. Lantus Optiset.

Insulin preparations available in UK

See Table 5.2.

Important practical points

Soluble/rapid-acting analogues

Soluble insulin is still recommended to be taken 30 min before meals, but there is no convincing evidence for the benefit of this, and patients frequently 'inject and eat'. However, soluble and premixed insulins containing soluble insulin should not be injected (or prescribed) after meals – surprisingly common.

Rapid-acting analogues have a faster onset of action than soluble insulin. The first to be introduced, insulin lispro in 1996, remains in monomeric form, and is therefore absorbed much quicker. Insulin aspart acts rapidly at the insulin receptor. Analogues and their mixtures (combined with isophane) are designed to be taken at the start of, during, or even shortly after meals. Patients (and carers) can therefore adjust doses of insulin according to how much has been eaten; they are useful when eating out, where food may arrive unpredictably, and are ideal for patients who take small supplementary doses of insulin with snacks. They reduce the incidence of post-meal hypoglycaemia, especially in the late morning. However, their relatively short duration of action means that they can wear off with consequent hyperglycaemia before the next meal if the interval between meals is >4–5 hours. This can be an advantage in the late evening where 'overlap' hypoglycaemia with bedtime isophane is potentially a problem; some patients use soluble insulin with breakfast and lunch, and a soluble analogue with the evening meal. Like all insulins, they suit some patients, but not others. Most clinical trials of these insulins show a small benefit in HbA_{1c} levels compared with isophane insulin, but these results conceal great variability in response between patients.

Conversion from soluble to rapid-acting analogue

Conversion is done unit for unit to begin with. In practice, patients appear to need higher doses of analogues than soluble for a given meal.

Intermediate-acting insulins (isophane, NPH)

These are still the most widely used background insulins, though their action is not long enough to be used as a once-daily insulin. Onset of action is gradual over 2–4 hours; this is useful if injection and meal times cannot be precisely coordinated, e.g. in the elderly receiving their insulin at home from community nursing teams. Peak action occurs around 6 hours after injection, so hypoglycaemia in the early hours of the morning is characteristic when given at bedtime as part of a basal-bolus regimen. For this reason they have been widely substituted with the long-acting analogues in type 1 patients (see below), but there is little evidence for inferiority of isophane/NPH insulin in type 2 diabetes.

The insulin is cloudy, and bottles and pens should be gently rolled or inverted up to 10 times before injection to homogenise the preparation.

Long-acting insulins

Long-acting (lente) and very-long-acting (ultralente) insulins have been withdrawn in the UK.

Long-acting analogues

Two are now in use – glargine (Lantus, Sanofi-Aventis) and detemir (Levemir, NovoNordisk). Their major advantage over isophane insulin is that they have a flat, almost peak-free action, lasting between 12 and 24 hours. Overnight hypoglycaemia is significantly reduced.

Glargine, introduced first, has a remarkably flat action, and clinically acts for 16–20 hours. Blood glucose levels change little overnight, so high pre-bedtime glucose levels may lead to similar high fasting levels the next day. This can be quite difficult to manage; a small dose of rapid-acting analogue taken with the bedtime dose of long-acting analogue might be useful.

Levemir was introduced in 2004. Its extended action is due to its tendency to self-associate into hexamers, its added fatty acid binding to albumin in the subcutaneous tissue, and albumin binding in the circulation (probably a minor effect). It is shorter acting than glargine and is best given twice daily. Both glargine and detemir are clear solutions. Like the short-acting analogues, they tend to show a statistical (though not clinically significant) benefit in HbA_{1c} reduction compared with isophane insulins. Slight weight loss has been demonstrated in clinical trials.

Conversion from isophane to long-acting analogue

Conversion is unit for unit. Careful monitoring of paired bedtime and fasting glucose levels is required. They cannot be mixed with other insulins, so patients on twice-daily free-mixed regimens will have to convert to a basal-bolus regimen.

When there is a problem with blood glucose control, the following practical points should be checked first:

- Type and dosage of insulin. If necessary this should be confirmed with a recent prescription, or preferably by checking the bottles, pens or cartridges themselves. Cartridges and needles should always be checked for compatibility with the specific pen types (only diabetes specialist nurses know about practical compatibilities). In the few people who now self-mix their insulins, technique should be carefully checked. Uniform mixing of cloudy insulin is important.
- Storage. Modern insulin has an effective shelf-life of about 2 years if kept refrigerated at 2–8° C, but storage in extreme tropical temperatures, hot car interiors, freezer compartments, and airplane holds is likely to cause denaturation. Manufacturers recommend storage for up to 4 weeks so long as temperatures are below 30° C.
- Injection sites. Lipoatrophy, probably an immune-mediated process, was usually associated with animal insulin, and is now

uncommon, but formation of fatty lumps (lipohypertrophy) is very common with non-analogue human insulins, if there are repeated injections over a long time into the same region – injections into these sites are less painful, but absorption can be very erratic. Even in the absence of clinical lipohypertrophy, absorption can be delayed from sites that have been injected frequently. There is a hint that soluble analogue insulins may not cause lipohypertrophy. Rotation of injection sites – thigh, buttock, abdomen (avoiding the immediate periumbilical area, which is the area many people associate with the 'abdomen') – should be encouraged. Injecting the upper arm should be avoided, which may result in intramuscular administration. Absorption is fastest and most consistent from the abdomen, and this is the preferred site for injection of pre-meal short-acting insulin.

- Injection technique. Fashions change, but the skin should be pinched and the injection given approximately perpendicular to the skin. Simple 'stabbing', which might not deliver into the subcutaneous tissue and is more likely to cause bruising, should be avoided. For most patients, 8 mm length pen needles are satisfactory; shorter needles should be reserved for children and very thin adults.

- Home blood glucose monitoring. Home blood glucose monitoring should be intensified temporarily, concentrating, as always, on times of day where blood glucose levels are at their most erratic. If instability overnight is suspected – as is likely, especially if using conventional isophane insulin – then a continuous glucose monitoring study is invaluable.

Insulin regimens

Twice-daily free mixture

This was the standard regimen for many years, but is much less commonly seen now in the UK, and is an unusual starting regimen. It is potentially very flexible, but in practice much less so. It is conventionally given as 2/3 isophane 1/3 soluble; 2/3 before breakfast, 1/3 before evening meal. If control is genuinely good, then there has to be a good reason for change from this regimen, but it is important to be aware of uniform doses (e.g. 20 units soluble with 20 units isophane twice daily), which patients tend to drift into. In these cases HbA_{1c} is unlikely to be good, but hypoglycaemia (especially nocturnal) is often not a problem, largely because the evening dose of isophane is too low.

Twice-daily fixed mixture (biphasic) insulin

This is a fixed proportion of soluble or rapid-acting analogue and isophane insulins (most popularly 30% soluble, 70% isophane, i.e. reflecting approximately the conventional 1/3, 2/3 split). It is convenient and in widespread use, especially in type 2 patients, but inflexible, and control is often suboptimal (typical HbA_{1c} ~8%). Rapid-acting analogue/isophane mixtures (NovoMix 30; Humalog Mix 25 and 50) have the advantage of the rapid-acting analogue component, in that they can be injected with or after a meal, but the convenience may not be reflected in consistently improved control compared with standard soluble/isophane mixtures.

Blood glucose levels around the middle of the day are often difficult to manage. Attempts to combat hyperglycaemia around lunchtime by increasing the morning dose may help, but it may also result in mid-morning hypoglycaemia as a result of the unwanted but inevitable increase in the dose of soluble/rapid-acting insulin. The best solution, if this is a continuing problem, is conversion to a basal-bolus regimen.

Other fixed mixtures containing 10, 20, 40 and 50% soluble insulin are still available, with the intention that the different mixtures could be used to manage differing meal sizes, and reduce post-prandial hypoglycaemia, but this nice theory did not work out in practice, and the 30 and 50% soluble (25% and 50% rapid-acting analogue) mixtures are now the major mixtures in current use.

The 50% mixtures (Mixtard 50, Humalog Mix50, Insuman Comb 50) are occasionally of use in patients taking a large breakfast or evening meal; they are especially useful in patients on nasogastric or PEG feeds (see Chapter 4).

In the UK they are overused in type 1 diabetes; they are useful for treatment in the period immediately after diagnosis, but all type 1 patients should be considered for intensive insulin treatment with a basal-bolus regimen.

Basal-bolus regimen

- Overnight isophane/overnight or morning long-acting analogue (glargine) or twice-daily long-acting analogue (detemir) with

- Three (or more) pre-prandial doses of soluble (or short-acting analogue).

These became practical in the mid-1980s with the introduction of pen devices that made it convenient to take insulin in the middle of the day. This regimen does not of itself improve glycaemic control, permit unrestricted eating or allow random mealtimes, but, used sensibly and flexibly, can lead to improved glycaemic control and patient satisfaction by allowing:

- meal times to be varied by 1–2 hours (especially important at lunchtime); and
- flexibility of meal sizes and physical activity.

It does not have demonstrable benefits in most overweight type 2 patients, but is the regimen of choice in the non-obese type 2 patient – who may have underlying late-onset type 1 diabetes.

It is argued (see above) whether this is a suitable regimen for newly diagnosed type 1 patients, but all young people should be given the opportunity of trying it as early as practicable, and certainly when moving to college or university, or when a home routine is otherwise likely to be disturbed.

Starting a basal-bolus regimen

Patients must be competent and reliable at monitoring blood glucose levels with a meter and recording and interpreting the results, to acquaint them with blood glucose responses to varying meals and activity.

If transferring from a twice-daily regimen, the total daily insulin dose should be reduced by ~10%; ~30–50% of the total daily dose is given as bedtime isophane or long-acting analogue, and the remainder divided between the three soluble or rapid-acting analogue doses. For example:

- twice-daily mixture: 28 units a.m., 20 units p.m. = 48 units
- deduct 10% = 5 units; remainder = 43 units
- pre-breakfast 6 units
- pre-lunch 8 units
- pre-evening meal 10 units
- bedtime isophane/long-acting analogue 18 units (~40% of total).

The regimen should always be started cautiously; hypoglycaemia weakens the patient's self-confidence, as well as their confidence in the regimen and in the person recommending it.

Other points

Development of a 'symmetrical/uniform' regimen

This results from patients trying to 'follow' blood glucose levels during the day without ensuring good fasting levels. Many of these patients have poor contacts with the hospital diabetes team. There is a risk of intermeal hypoglycaemia, but as with the uniform free-mixing regimen, patients are often protected against this by the high fasting glucose levels resulting from inadequate bedtime isophane.

Pre-meal doses rarely need to be more than 10–14 units (1 U $\cong$ 10 g carbohydrate), but very high carbohydrate meals are likely to require more – and the doses of fast-acting analogues also tend to be higher.

Some conscientious patients take additional small doses of insulin before snacks, and if fast-acting analogues are being used, then additional doses with, for example, a dessert after a long meal, would be appropriate.

A regimen frequently used in Europe modifies the standard basal-bolus regimen by adding in a further small dose of isophane insulin in the morning, giving true basal insulin during the day. This will become less common with the increasing use of glargine, but detemir, which is best given twice daily, fits neatly into this scheme.

Continuous subcutaneous insulin infusion (CSII)

CSII was popular in the 1970s–1980s, and is now in standard use in most countries as a result of innovations in technology that have improved the reliability (and reduced the size) of the pumps, and of a reasonable amount of evidence that in selected groups of type 1 patients it can significantly improve glycaemic control.

The principle is that a soluble (or more commonly now rapid-acting) analogue is delivered continuously as a background (basal) dose (around 1 unit/h) from a portable infusion pump into the subcutaneous tissue of the abdomen, through a small indwelling plastic catheter. Prandial doses similar to those used in a basal-bolus regimen can be delivered from the pump on top of the background dose. Pumps and peripherals are moderately costly (around £100 a month; CSII has been endorsed by NICE, though funding in the UK is still a major problem) and 24-hour support from a dedicated and trained team is mandatory for safety and optimum results.

Ketoacidosis resulting from pump failure was a fear with early models, but sophisticated alarm procedures have largely removed this complication. Skin infections at the catheter insertion site occur, but cellulitis and abscess formation are uncommon.

CSII should be considered in:

- motivated patients keen on preventing, or who have already, early microvascular complications
- erratic blood glucose control with frequent hypoglycaemic and/or hyperglycaemic episodes
- pregnancy or pre-pregnancy where rapid control has to be established
- 'brittle diabetes'; though this indication requires careful consideration of any underlying psychological problems
- insulin-resistant patients (daily requirement >100 units insulin).

There are occasional reports of benefit in extremely insulin-resistant type 2 diabetes where all attempts at control have been to no avail. Even where overall control cannot be markedly improved, quality of life can be significantly improved.

This is an intermediate-level technique that should be available widely to a larger number of patients in the UK. Adequate motivation, together with a desire or need for overall better control, should be sufficient to guarantee at least a trial.

Management of problems with insulin regimens

Fasting hyperglycaemia

Unexpected fasting hyperglycaemia (CBG >10 mmol/L) or high variability of fasting glucose levels in the presence of otherwise good daytime glucose control is common. The introduction of continuous glucose monitoring, where available, has made the analysis of the problem much easier, and the introduction of long-acting analogues has improved the management of erratic overnight control. There are three possible reasons:

- Somogyi phenomenon: nocturnal hypoglycaemia → secretion of counter-regulatory hormones → insulin resistance → 'rebound' hyperglycaemia. Even the existence of this phenomenon was doubted by some, but at least in terms of glucose levels monitored with CGMS, it appears to be frequent

- dawn phenomenon: rising blood glucose levels between 05:00 and 08:00 h due to delayed insulin resistance caused by normal surges of growth hormone that occur during sleep. Probably a minor effect
- declining insulin levels from isophane injection given the previous evening/before bed (operationally this seems to be rather uncommon).

Nocturnal hypoglycaemia

This is common, possibly almost invariable, with isophane insulin taken as a mixture with the evening meal or at bedtime as part of a basal-bolus regimen. CGMS has revealed that it is nearly always asymptomatic – patients remain asleep, and counter-regulation occurs, though sometimes not for up to 2–4 hours. Severe nocturnal hypoglycaemia is a likely cause of the 'dead in bed' syndrome (an otherwise well, usually young diabetic person is found dead in the morning in an undisturbed bed).

The effect of alcohol should be remembered: initial hyperglycaemia, followed by hypoglycaemia (though this is not always the pattern found), usually in the middle of the night after an evening drinking. This is an important education point for all insulin-taking diabetic patients.

Clinical approach

Patients taking fixed mixture with their evening meal
The evening dose is split into soluble/rapid-acting analogue with the evening meal, and isophane (or preferably long-acting analogue) at bedtime. This can be done strictly on the basis of the pre-existing split, e.g. Humalog Mix25, 24 units with evening meal → Humalog 6 units with evening meal (be prepared to increase this in accordance with post-meal monitoring) + ~18–20 units glargine or detemir.

Patients taking basal-bolus regimen
If patients are taking soluble insulin and eating late in the evening, then taking their bedtime isophane 1–2 hours later, overlap hypoglycaemia in the early hours can occur. The evening meal insulin should be changed to a rapid-acting analogue, and consideration given to changing the bedtime insulin to a long-acting analogue.

New developments

Inhaled insulin preparations are a highly logical approach to taking rapid-acting insulin, with the possibility of longer-acting agents becoming available in due course. However, the development of inhaled insulin, which started in the early 1990s, has had some technological (inhaler) and biological problems (effect of insulin on pulmonary function, and vice versa; effect of pulmonary function, for example during upper respiratory tract infection and in smokers, on insulin absorption). Having resolved these problems, several systems are in development, and will come to market over the next 1–2 years. The benefits of injection-free administration are apparent, but widespread education will be required to overcome the natural reluctance of some patients to move to a completely different mode of administration.

Buccal, transdermal and oral insulin preparations are currently in development

6 PERIOPERATIVE MANAGEMENT

Metabolic responses to surgery

In diabetic patients, surgery induces insulin resistance through several mechanisms. There is increased secretion of counter-regulatory hormones, especially catecholamines, cortisol and growth hormone. Catecholamines themselves inhibit insulin secretion; the combination of insulin resistance and reduced insulin secretion, together with perioperative starvation, results in:

- increased lipolysis and ketogenesis
- increased protein breakdown
- hyperglycaemia.

Although it is difficult to demonstrate any differences in wound healing in people with diabetes, postoperative infections are more common in poorly controlled diabetes (see Chapter 8), at least in part as a result of defective neutrophil function.

Management of diabetes in surgical patients

The aims of perioperative diabetic management are to avoid:

- excess mortality and morbidity, especially through infection
- severe hyperglycaemia
- ketoacidosis in type 1 patients
- hypoglycaemia during anaesthesia.

Preoperative diabetic control

Increasing use of minimally invasive and day-case surgery means that patients are less likely to be admitted preoperatively for glycaemic stabilisation. It is therefore important that glycaemic control is optimised before admission.

It should be recognised, however, that mean HbA_{1c} level in a hospital diabetic clinic is ~8%. Improving on this in many individuals may be difficult, and probably has little impact on perioperative complications. Try to improve HbA_{1c} levels of 9% or more, representing mean diurnal blood glucose levels ≥ 12–13 mmol/L. However, some patients are chronically in very poor control; a decision must be taken whether or not to go ahead with surgery, balancing risks and benefits. Indefinite or recurrent postponement pending improved control in these patients is dispiriting for everyone, and this is the group likely to benefit from a few days of intensive in-patient preoperative management. Recall that certain surgically treatable conditions, for example cataract, may themselves hinder improved control.

Day-case surgery is possible in insulin-treated patients, but they must be in good control, carefully self-monitoring, and should be first on the operating list – with very careful perioperative monitoring. Most insulin-treated patients will require admission 24 hours preoperatively. During this period, 7-point blood glucose series should be obtained (before meals, 2 hours after meals and at bedtime) while on the patient's usual insulin regimen. If there is enough time, change temporarily to a basal-bolus regimen if control is very poor, but attempts may make things worse in the short term. In very poorly controlled patients, an intravenous insulin infusion might be wise.

Patients with diabetes, especially those taking insulin, should be placed first on an operating list, a sensible rule that is increasingly not observed. This places patients at increased risk because of the need for prolonged insulin infusions and because they are more likely to return from theatre late in the day.

Late diabetic complications in relation to surgery are:

- coronary artery disease and congestive heart failure (ECG, CXR)
- diabetic nephropathy (anaemia, fluid overload, acute on chronic renal failure)
- diabetic foot ulcers (underlying osteomyelitis, MRSA status, systemic sepsis)
- advanced autonomic neuropathy (increased risk of perioperative cardiovascular events, possibly as a result of arrhythmias or prolonged QT_c interval); postural blood pressure drop and RR interval variation to deep breathing (see Chapter 11).

These patients should be managed very closely with anaesthetists.

Summary of perioperative management

See Table 6.1.

Table 6.1 Summary of perioperative management

	Minor procedures	Other surgery
Diet-controlled	No special precautions if well controlled	Avoid i.v. dextrose Monitor CBG regularly during surgery If CBG consistently >12, consider GIK infusion Do not assume diet-treated patients are well controlled
Tablet-treated type 2	Omit medication on morning of surgery (omit glibenclamide the previous evening) Operate in morning where possible Monitor blood glucose 2-hourly Restart medication when patient eating and drinking	Omit medication on morning of surgery (omit glibenclamide the previous evening) Start GIK infusion by 08:00 Continue postop until patient eating May need s.c. insulin (basal-bolus) for a few days until oral therapy restarted
Insulin-treated (type 1 and 2)	If very short procedure, omit insulin while nil by mouth, monitor CBG before and after procedure and restart insulin when eating. Closely supervised, this regimen can also be used for other day-case procedures in well-controlled insulin-treated patients, provided procedure is first on the list, patients can be monitored carefully during the day, and are not discharged home alone	Use GIK/Alberti regimen (see below)

Insulin regimens for perioperative care

Single bag infusion (GIK, Alberti regime)

This is the safest regimen, and is suitable for most surgery. Use of a 10% dextrose solution is probably best as it limits the volume of fluid if the regimen has to be administered over a long period. The fluid volume must be taken into account in perioperative care, but other fluids can be co-administered as required.

- Add 15 units soluble insulin (Actrapid/Humulin S) and 10 mmol KCl to 500 mL 10% dextrose and infuse at 100 mL/h.
- Preoperatively, measure blood glucose hourly; the infusion can be altered to 20 units if CBG >11 mmol/L, or to 10 units if CBG <6 mmol/L.
- If CBG <5 mmol/L, stop the infusion for 20–30 minutes, and restart if CBG >6 mmol/L.
- Postoperatively, measure CBG hourly for the first 6 hours, then 4-hourly if blood glucose levels are stable.
- Stop food and usual insulin when the infusion is started. When the patient is eating again, give normal pre-prandial insulin, and discontinue the infusion 30 minutes later.

Continuous variable intravenous insulin infusion

Infuse soluble insulin via a syringe pump – 50 units soluble insulin (Actrapid/Humulin S) in 50 mL 0.9% saline in a 50 mL syringe.

Use this regimen:

- for emergency surgery when complicated by a hyperglycaemic state
- when there is concern about the stability of the diabetes
- when there is concern about the fluid status of the patient, e.g. cardiac or renal impairment. There is no need to use the above regimen for most routine surgery, as it is complex, and requires intensive nursing and medical supervision – hourly CBG measurements are mandatory. The i.v. insulin must be run together with intravenous 5% or 10% dextrose, to avoid the risk of hypoglycaemia. Watch for hypokalaemia.

Use the initial infusion rates shown in Table 6.2, depending on blood glucose levels, and measure CBG every hour until stable levels are achieved (then every 2–4 hours).

Table 6.2 Variable insulin infusion

Blood glucose (mmol/L)	Insulin infusion rate (units [mL]/h)
0–4	0
4.1–7.0	1
7.1–11.0	2
11.1–17.0	4
17.1–22.0	6
>22	8 (review regimen)

Insulin requirements vary between and within subjects according to various factors, especially those that increase insulin resistance. Always be prepared to adjust a fixed regimen according to blood glucose monitoring results.

Perfect glycaemic control (4–7 mmol/L) is neither easily achievable, especially in the postoperative period, nor desirable, in view of the risk of hypoglycaemia. Where intensive control is required (e.g. post-cardiac surgery) patients should be managed in a PCU/ITU environment. Until there is definitive evidence of benefit for tighter control in general surgical cases, CBG levels up to 10–12 mmol/L are satisfactory, and short-term mild hyperglycaemia is preferable to hypoglycaemia.

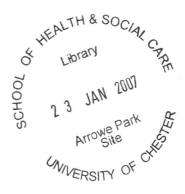

7 MANAGEMENT OF TYPE 2 DIABETES

Insulin resistance as well as deteriorating β-cell function are the two major targets of management of type 2 diabetes. Sites of action of some agents used in management of type 2 diabetes are indicated in the filled boxes in Figure 7.1.

Most cases of type 2 diabetes are diagnosed and managed in primary care, and the emphasis is increasingly on management in the community (see Chapter 14). However, newly diagnosed type 2 patients are frequently seen in A&E, or are found on routine in- or out-patient screening; for example, up to 50% of acute coronary syndrome patients

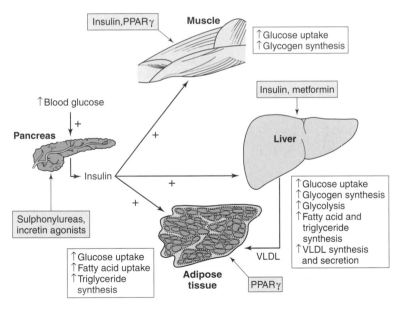

Figure 7.1 Effects of insulin on the important tissues, especially liver, muscle and adipose tissue. Insulin resistance at these sites is the hallmark of type 2 diabetes throughout the course of the disease.

have a previously undiagnosed significant abnormality of glucose tolerance, either IGT or frank diabetes (see Chapter 4). When incidentally found, for example in A&E, unless there is an associated hyperglycaemic emergency, or ≥2+ ketonuria on urinalysis, these patients do not usually require admission – but there must be a firm plan in place for their rapid assessment and follow-up with their primary care team.

At least 20% of type 2 patients have microvascular complications at diagnosis, most commonly retinopathy and microalbuminuria. A similar proportion has subclinical or clinical macrovascular disease, as a result of the preceding 20 or more years of insulin resistance/metabolic syndrome. Detection and management of complications at diagnosis is just as important as achieving impeccable glycaemic control.

Initial examination should include:

- urinalysis for protein and ketones
- dilated fundoscopy, especially for maculopathy, or formal review with an optometrist
- clinical examination for peripheral vascular disease and neuropathy.

Laboratory tests:

- creatinine + electrolytes, HbA_{1c}
- thyroid function (note high prevalence of subclinical hypothyroidism – up to 1 in 12 – in white female type 2 diabetic patients)
- ECG.

Although liver functions and fasting lipids are invariably measured, they (and urinary albumin excretion) are likely to be abnormal depending on the degree of hyperglycaemia and underlying metabolic syndrome. They are more reliably measured about 3 months after diagnosis. Although most of these patients will have 'ordinary' type 2 diabetes, always bear in mind:

- pancreatic causes, especially alcohol, and underlying pancreatic carcinoma
- genetic haemochromatosis
- whether it is actually late-onset type 1 diabetes (LADA) – see below and Chapter 1
- syndromic type 2 diabetes (see Chapter 1), suggested by:
  - multisystem involvement
  - family history of diabetes/deafness

- first-cousin parents
- insulin resistance in the absence of obesity.

All patients must see at or shortly after diagnosis:

- a dietician
- a nurse practitioner/practice nurse/community diabetes specialist nurse
- a chiropodist.

The general clinical approach to the newly diagnosed type 2 patient

Patients who are only slightly overweight before diagnosis (e.g. BMI <28) may have late-onset type 1 diabetes, and must be supervised very carefully. They often show a good initial response to sulphonylureas (see below) but control may subsequently deteriorate rapidly. Any patient with persistent 1+ or more ketonuria, especially if there is weight loss or failure to regain lost weight with OHAs, should be considered to have type 1 diabetes, and needs insulin treatment soon. GAD antibody status (see Chapter 1) may be helpful in confirming immune-mediated diabetes.

Assess all patients for the components of the insulin resistance syndrome (see Chapter 2) and the presence of macrovascular disease. This is more important in prognosis than excessive concern with achieving normal blood glucose levels immediately. Patients should be persuaded that a true multimodal approach to their condition (along the lines of the Steno type 2 study, 2003) will reap greater benefits than striving merely for near-normoglycaemia. Weight loss, attention to dietary components, and regular activity go without saying, yet are often neglected in favour of quick fixes with oral hypoglycaemic agents.

However, severely symptomatic overweight patients, e.g. with random glucose levels >15 mmol/L, should be considered for short-term treatment with a low-dose sulphonylurea, as it will at least initially produce a good clinical effect. Low-dose metformin, which should be the mainstay of treatment in such patients, and should be thought of as a disease-modifying drug rather than just an oral hypoglycaemic agent, should be started immediately, with the aim of withdrawing the sulphonylurea and maintaining the patient on metformin alone. The traditional approach of 3 months diet, then consideration of metformin, is not rational in the light of the UKPDS results.

The place of the anti-obesity agents orlistat and sibutramine is still not clear. In randomised controlled trials (RCTs) up to a year both agents are effective (sibutramine 10–15 mg daily reduces weight by ~6–8 kg, with a fall in HbA_{1c} ~0.5–1.0%; orlistat 120 mg t.d.s. causes slightly less weight loss, ~3–5 kg over the same period) and in clinical practice they are also effective when used as part of a comprehensive weight-management programme. Where this is not available, success is more limited; the fat malabsorption induced by orlistat hinders compliance in the early stages of treatment, and although in general better tolerated, sibutramine causes slight but significant elevations in blood pressure, which nevertheless in RCTs are generally easily treated. Orlistat may have a role in delaying progression of IGT to diabetes (see Chapter 2).

Oral hypoglycaemic agents

Individual response varies, the response is related to the initial level of glycaemia, and reductions in HbA_{1c} quoted in placebo-controlled RCTs are greater than can be expected in clinical practice (see Table 7.1). This is because patients are generally supervised more closely in RCTs than in clinical practice, and because HbA_{1c} tends to rise in placebo-treated patients – results are usually quoted as the difference between the drug and placebo responses.

Table 7.1   Expected reductions in HbA_{1c} with various OHAs

Drug	Reduction in HbA_{1c} (%)
Sulphonylureas and meglitinides	1.5–2.0
Metformin	0.8–2.0
Sulphonylurea + metformin	Up to 2.5
Acarbose	0.4–0.7
Glitazones	0.6–1.2

Metformin

Action

Metformin has peripheral effects only (it does not stimulate pancreatic insulin secretion); it increases muscle glucose uptake and metabolism (not consistently demonstrated), decreases hepatic gluconeogenesis, and has minor but beneficial effects on:

- lipids (significant only in people with very poor initial glycaemic control)
- blood pressure (contentious)
- coagulation factors
- weight – UKPDS showed that it does not cause weight loss (still widely and wrongly believed), but there is modest and stable weight gain (around 2 kg) – though this should be compared with the mean 5 kg weight gain in patients treated with sulphonylureas or insulin.

Intensive metformin treatment in obese patients (mean BMI 31) was associated with decreased risk of myocardial infarction in UKPDS. This benefit appears to have been maintained in the 5-year post-UKPDS follow-up. It is safe and effective in adult doses in children with type 2 diabetes.

Dose

Metformin is effective in the dose range 500–2000 mg daily, with reductions in fasting glucose of 1–4 mmol/L over this range, and corresponding HbA_{1c} reductions of 0.8–2.0%. There is little evidence for increased efficacy at doses >2 g/day, and side-effects are more common. At its highest dose it is as effective as any other treatment used in type 2 diabetes – it is not a 'weak' agent. It is therefore effective at the lowest dose of 500 mg/day (HbA_{1c} fall ~0.5%), so even if patients can only tolerate this small dose (given with the main meal of the day) then it will confer some benefit. The modified-release preparation, with once-daily dosing, may aid compliance and reduce side-effects.

Metformin should be taken with meals, starting at 500 mg once or twice daily, and titrated to maximum effect. Gastrointestinal side-effects (diarrhoea, nausea, dyspepsia and flatulence) are common in the first 1–2 weeks, but <5% of patients cannot tolerate metformin at any dose. In clinical practice delayed side-effects are occasionally seen, even after quite long periods during which metformin has apparently been well tolerated. If these symptoms occur, the patient should be observed for a short time after withdrawal of metformin before embarking on gastrointestinal investigations.

Contraindications

Renal impairment is the main concern; conventionally, serum creatinine >120 μmol/L has been considered a contraindication to metformin treatment. A more recent general consensus is that it can be used safely so long as serum creatinine is <~150 μmol/L (or more precisely if creatinine clearance is >30 mL/min). Thereafter it should be withdrawn (and used with caution if creatinine clearance is between 30 and 50 mL/min). The potency of this agent should not be underestimated, and alternative strategies must be in place when it is withdrawn (this will usually be insulin treatment). The clinical impression is that HbA_{1c} levels can rise by up to 2–3% when a substantial dose of metformin is withdrawn in people with moderately impaired renal function.

Severe hepatic impairment, and heart failure that is not under good control, are both contraindications to metformin treatment. Mildly abnormal liver function tests, very common in people with diabetes as a result of NAFLD, are not a contraindication, and metformin may well improve the results. There is an erroneous view that metformin is contraindicated in patients who have had a myocardial infarction; other than the general precautions, the UKPDS results suggest the converse, that patients with established coronary artery disease should generally be treated with metformin (see glitazones), and it should not be withdrawn if insulin treatment is started (see below).

Lactic acidosis and vitamin B_{12} levels
Lactic acidosis is much feared, but nowadays is an extremely rare complication of metformin treatment, usually occurring in the presence of several concomitant contraindications. Despite several studies showing subtle impairment of vitamin B_{12} metabolism in long-term metformin treatment, serum B_{12} levels remain normal; routine measurements are not required. Macrocytosis or low B_{12} levels in type 2 patients on metformin should therefore be investigated in the usual way.

Radiological contrast medium-induced lactic acidosis
The conventional view is that metformin should be withheld 48 hours before and after a procedure involving intravenous contrast agent, because of the increased risk of lactic acidosis (both agents are excreted unchanged via the kidneys). In practice, such cases nearly always occur in patients with impaired renal function, and stopping metformin before the procedure is more difficult than discontinuing it afterwards. Where possible, review previous laboratory results to establish any trends in renal function.

- In patients with normal renal function (serum creatinine <130 μmol/L) metformin does not need to be withheld, but adequate hydration should always be ensured.

- Where there is renal impairment, metformin should be withheld for 48 hours after the procedure. Most patients will not need alternative diabetes treatment over this period. Adequate peri-procedural hydration should be ensured and renal function checked before restarting metformin.

Sulphonylureas and meglitinides (prandial insulin releasers)

Table 7.2 Sulphonylureas and meglitinides

Drug	Effect duration (h)	Daily dose range (mg)	Max effective dose (mg)	Dosages/ day	Comments
Sulphonylureas					
Glibenclamide (USA: glyburide)	20–24	2.5–20	10	1–2	No longer a first-line agent
Gliclazide	10–15	40–320	160	1 up to 160 mg; higher doses divided	m/r (once-daily) available, dose range 30–90 mg (≅80–240 mg non-m/r gliclazide)
Glipizide	12–14	2.5–40	20	1 up to 15 mg; higher doses divided	m/r available in USA
Glimepiride	24	1–6	4	1 at all doses	
Meglitinides					
Repaglinide	Few	1.5–16	16	0.5–4 mg with each meal	Take 15–30 min before main meals
Nateglinide	Few	180–540	540	60–180 mg with each meal	Take 15–30 min before main meals; licensed in combination with metformin, not as monotherapy

m/r, modified-release.

The sulphonylureas have been workhorses of diabetes therapy for more than 50 years. The meglitinides, which operate through similar mechanisms, have been introduced over the past 7 years. Neither should be used as first-line treatments in overweight or obese patients, or those with multiple insulin resistance characteristics, where metformin is mandatory.

Action

The sulphonylureas stimulate first- and second-phase pancreatic insulin secretion, by binding to the sulphonylurea receptor on the β-cell. This closes the Kir 6.2 potassium channel, resulting in calcium influx, stimulating insulin secretion. The meglitinides bind to a different site of the sulphonylurea receptor, and have a much more rapid onset and offset of action. They are therefore suitable for taking immediately before a meal, for controlling predominant post-prandial hyperglycaemia, and in patients prone to hypoglycaemia with standard sulphonylureas.

Some sulphonylureas, especially glibenclamide, cross-react with and close cardiac potassium channels and reduce protective ischaemic preconditioning. Whether this is of clinical significance is not known, but concern persists, and glibenclamide, especially as it is long-acting, and carries an increased risk of hypoglycaemia, should probably be considered outdated. Other sulphonylureas, including gliclazide and glimepiride, and the meglitinides, do not have this potential adverse effect.

Doses should be low initially, increasing in accordance with blood glucose monitoring. Dose–response relationships for the sulphonylureas are weak, and there may be decreasing effectiveness at very high doses. Since they are most often useful in the early stages of diabetes, when β-cell function is better preserved, the common practice of increasing sulphonylurea dosage in patients with long-standing diabetes in the hope of delaying additional therapy is not rational. There is increasing evidence that sulphonylurea failure begins after about 6 months, and is progressive.

Additional effects

Sulphonylureas and meglitinides have no significant effects on insulin resistance, surrogate indicators of insulin resistance, or lipids and, therefore, unlike metformin or the glitazones, are probably not disease-modifying agents. Because of their primary pancreatic effect, they are therefore of greatest value in the relatively small proportion of type 2 patients with absent insulin-resistant characteristics; some of these will have late-onset type 1 diabetes, so failure to respond, or weakening of the effect after 12–24 months should be looked for. Glitazones would be considered sound second-line agents in insulin-resistant type 2 patients.

Weight gain
Weight gain can be substantial with the standard sulphonylureas (the UKPDS reported a mean weight gain of 2.3 kg), but may be less with the meglitinides.

Sulphonylurea-induced hypoglycaemia
Hypoglycaemia can occur with any sulphonylurea (0.4–0.6% /year in the UKPDS), and is not unknown with the meglitinides. Glibenclamide is the main culprit; even though it is long-acting, glimepiride appears to carry a lower risk of hypoglycaemia, especially in the elderly.

Hypoglycaemia characteristically occurs about 4 hours after a dose, commonly at the end of the morning, particularly after mild exertion and omitting any mid-morning snack, e.g. on shopping or golfing mornings. Patients should be taught to recognise the symptoms of hypoglycaemia, as there is a widespread belief that only people taking insulin experience hypoglycaemia.

Profound and prolonged hypoglycaemia can occur in:

- the elderly
- those with intercurrent illness, malnutrition or alcoholism
- those with impaired renal function.

Admit, especially the elderly, and treat with a prolonged infusion of 10–20% glucose. Bolus injections of glucose, and of glucagon, will stimulate residual insulin secretion in type 2 patients, hence the need for continuing glucose infusion with careful monitoring. Potassium levels, which may fall under the influence of high insulin levels, should be monitored. Octreotide might be of value in very severe and prolonged cases.

Thiazolidinediones (glitazones, TZDs)

Thiazolidinediones are an important group of drugs. The prototype, troglitazone, was introduced briefly in the UK during 1997, but withdrawn because of rare but serious hepatic side-effects. It was withdrawn in the USA in 2000. The two successor compounds, rosiglitazone and pioglitazone, introduced in 2000, have no adverse hepatic effects.

Action

Glitazones are PPARγ (peroxisome proliferator-activated receptor gamma) agonists, acting at nuclear receptors to stimulate various insulin-sensitive genes. They have multiple actions in major insulin-sensitive tissues – muscle, liver and adipose tissue – for example, increasing glucose uptake, decreasing gluconeogenesis and glycogenolysis; increasing fatty acid uptake, lipogenesis and differentiation of adipocytes. Like metformin, they require insulin to produce glucose-lowering effects and, like metformin, they are antihyperglycaemic, rather than hypoglycaemic, so carry a low risk of hypoglycaemia when used as monotherapy. They reduce insulin resistance, and also probably have some preservative β-cell effect. Although they would appear to be more useful in those with phenotypic features of insulin resistance, clinically this is not necessarily the case, and responsiveness to the glitazones cannot be predicted on simple clinical grounds. Carefully observed therapeutic trials in individual patients are therefore important with this group of drugs. Onset of blood glucose lowering is slow and does not maximise until 2–4 months after starting treatment, so they should not be used as initial therapy in symptomatically hyperglycaemic newly diagnosed patients.

Additional effects

Glitazones have been shown to have a range of non-glucose effects that make them potentially beneficial in reducing macrovascular events in type 2 diabetes. These include a small blood pressure lowering effect, and a generally beneficial effect on lipid profiles (pioglitazone reduces triglycerides and elevates HDL, while rosiglitazone slightly elevates LDL levels, though this may be in the more buoyant, less atherogenic fraction: see Chapter 13). There are also effects on inflammatory markers, e.g. white cell count, hsCRP and microalbuminuria, and both agents reduce carotid artery intima-media thickness (see below). The PROactive study (pioglitazone) – secondary prevention in patients with type 2 diabetes and ischaemic heart disease – reported positively in 2005, showing a significant 16% risk reduction in all cause mortality/non-fatal MI/stroke in patients treated with pioglitazone 45 mg daily for about 3 years, in addition to all other treatment (including insulin). This is the first compelling evidence in a large scale RCT that a medication for diabetes can reduce macrovascular risk. There is also suggestive evidence that rosiglitazone reduces the risk of restenosis after coronary stenting in diabetic patients. Although caution is always required in interpreting results that claim effects beyond blood glucose lowering, it appears that the glitazones may have an important role in patients with ischaemic heart disease, as is the case with metformin. Primary prevention data on glitazones and macrovascular disease will be available over the next few years.

Adverse effects

- Weight gain, largely adipose, can be substantial (2–6 kg), but several studies have shown that this is associated with a reduction in intra-abdominal fat, and redistribution to less metabolically active sites. Mild ankle oedema is common, but rarely troublesome.
- Exacerbation of heart failure: use with great care in patients with heart failure (though where they are used, it appears that overall mortality is improved; the same appears to be the case with metformin).
- Anaemia: Haemoglobin fall is usually around 1 g/dl, sometimes greater; this is of little significance in the non-anaemic patient, but anaemia is common and occurs early in diabetic renal failure (see Chapter 10), a scenario where substitution of a glitazone for discontinued metformin is likely. The mechanism of the anaemia is not clear.
- Not to be used in patients with impaired liver function, e.g. ALT >2.5× ULN (around 85 iU/L in most laboratories; to be discontinued if ALT is consistently >3× ULN).

The requirement for liver functions to be monitored every 2 months has been lifted; baseline LFTs, with repeat measurements as clinically indicated, are now recommended. In many cases transaminases, alkaline phosphatase and γGT levels fall with glitazone treatment, consistent with improvement in hepatic insulin resistance and consequent non-alcoholic fatty liver disease – but there are no studies that confirm improvement in hepatic histology in patients with only slightly abnormal LFTs.

Agents

- Rosiglitazone: 4 mg, 8 mg.
- Pioglitazone: 15 mg, 30 mg, 45 mg.

Various fixed-dose combinations of metformin and rosiglitazone (Avandamet) may aid compliance (e.g. metformin 1 g + rosiglitazone 2 mg or 4 mg b.d.), in patients taking maximum metformin and requiring a second agent. Similar combination preparations of pioglitazone and metformin (ACTOplus met), containing metformin 500 or 850 mg + pioglitazone 15 mg have been approved in the USA.

Monotherapy
Both glitazones are licensed for monotherapy. In practice, this means use in patients who cannot tolerate metformin at any dose or in whom it is contraindicated (usually renal impairment), and for whom a sulphonylurea is not thought advisable – for example, people with likely metabolic syndrome.

Dual oral therapy
Both agents are licensed for use with metformin, and this is their main indication:

- in patients not achieving target HbA_{1c} on maximum tolerated metformin monotherapy
- in other high risk groups, where insulin resistance is likely to be important, e.g. in ethnic minority patients, those with coronary artery disease.

Triple oral therapy (glitazone + metformin + sulphonylurea)
Rosiglitazone is now licensed for use in triple therapy, though it has been used off license in this way for several years as an 'insulin-sparing' or 'insulin-deferring' agent. This speculative use has now been confirmed in the PROactive study (see below). Interestingly, the response to this treatment (addition of a glitazone to sulphonylurea + maximum metformin) is not related to known duration of diabetes, nor to any specific clinical or biochemical measure. It is therefore a useful strategy before considering insulin therapy in all patients who are not obviously insulin deficient, and perhaps especially where there is concern about poor long-term glycaemic response to insulin treatment, for example in the overweight.

Glycaemic benefit
Variable, and not predictable on clinical or biochemical grounds, though there generally appears to be a better response in patients with a short duration of diabetes. Between 60 and 90% of patients respond (e.g. HbA_{1c} falls >1.0% after 4 months). In an RCT of triple therapy with

rosiglitazone, mean fall was 0.4% (4 mg daily) and 0.8% (8 mg daily). In individuals with very poor glycaemic control e.g. HbA_{1c} 9–12%, sustained falls of 2–3% are not unusual, though there is an association between weight gain and glycaemic improvement. Patients who do not respond after 4–6 months should be considered for insulin treatment. Occasional hypoglycaemia, presumably due to persisting sulphonylurea therapy, occurs, usually when HbA_{1c} falls to <6.5% or thereabouts, and some patients are eventually maintained on a combination of glitazone + metformin. Glycaemic control appears to remain stable for up to 2–3 years in patients who respond (compare sulphonylureas). There is increasing evidence that the vascular benefits of glitazones (e.g. in reducing carotid intima-media thickness) are independent of glycaemic response, so there is a good case at present for maintaining glitazone treatment in patients who do not have a significant glycaemic response, especially if they have established macrovascular disease.

Glitazones and insulin

Pioglitazone is currently licensed in the USA in combination with insulin, but not in the UK. The combination appears to carry an increased risk of rapid weight gain and fluid retention, but not of heart failure. There is a case for its use under careful supervision in secondary care in patients who, despite insulin treatment, continue to have poor or very poor glycaemic control, and who have progressive microvascular complications or established macrovascular disease. The combination appears to carry less risk of side-effects if the dose of insulin is lower – and many patients on large doses of insulin (>100 U/day) can gradually reduce the dose without adversely affecting glycaemic control. In patients who respond, hypoglycaemia, requiring further reductions in insulin, is not uncommon. PROactive (see above) convincingly showed that pioglitazone 45 mg daily reduced the need for insulin treatment by about 50% over 3 years, while also showing that HbA_{1c} could be improved consistently by ~0.5% over the same period when added to any regimen, including the 30% already taking insulin.

α-Glucosidase inhibitors

Action

These drugs inhibit enzymes that break down polysaccharides and sucrose in the small intestine, leading to delayed absorption of glucose, and lower post-prandial glucose peaks – though the total amount of glucose absorbed is unchanged. There are changes in secretion of incretins (e.g. $\downarrow$GIP, $\uparrow$GLP-1), but overall insulin secretion is reduced. Their effects are most marked in patients taking a high complex carbohydrate diet.

Acarbose was used in a limb of the UKPDS, where it was shown to reduce HbA_{1c} levels by around 0.5%. This relatively weak effect, together with its marked gastrointestinal side effects, especially flatulence, limited its use of late; however, the STOP-NIDDM trial (2002) showed it had a powerful effect in reducing progression of IGT to type 2 diabetes, but only while the drug was being taken. It also reduced the incidence of macrovascular events and of new hypertension, though these outcomes have been challenged. Overall, this group of drugs should probably be used again more, especially in early type 2 diabetes in the primary care setting.

Some patients can tolerate the combination of metformin and an α-glucosidase inhibitor.

Dose escalation should be slow, e.g. acarbose 50 mg with main meal, increasing to 50 mg t.d.s. Maximum dose is 100 mg t.d.s. (occasionally associated with abnormal liver functions, so should be monitored when used in high doses).

Insulin treatment in type 2 diabetes

Insulin deficiency can be demonstrated at the time of diagnosis of type 2 diabetes, and proceeds linearly. It is generally thought that at the time maximum OHAs (sulphonylurea + metformin) begin to fail (HbA_{1c} >8.0% around 10 years after diagnosis), insulin deficiency predominates over insulin resistance. Clinically, however, this may not be the case, especially in overweight patients. Insulin treatment often does not result in as low HbA_{1c} levels as in type 1 patients, and clinically insulin resistance still seems to be a major problem.

Non-overweight patients (BMI <28)

These patients, many of whom will have late-onset type 1 diabetes, should be prioritised for insulin treatment when maximum OHAs fail; in RCTs, most patients at this stage have average HbA_{1c} levels ~9.0–9.5%, so intervention is often late. Weight gain is relatively small, and with intensified insulin, as in type 1 diabetes, good glycaemic control can be anticipated.

Overweight patients

These patients are still a major management dilemma, source of contention and subject of partisan disputes. Small but carefully conducted RCTs in the early 1990s showed that insulin treatment, using any regimen, in overweight patients failed to sustain glycaemic improvements beyond 12 months. This was confirmed in the UKPDS. Few RCTs last more than 6 months, and this duration must be considered inadequate where treatment is likely to be lifelong. UKPDS confirmed that insulin treatment conferred no glycaemic advantage over any other treatment modality in the long term and therefore no advantage in terms of prevention or slowing progression of microvascular complications. Hypoglycaemia is common, and weight gain substantial (about 5 kg, slightly less with basal insulin + OHAs), exacerbating several features of the metabolic syndrome ($\uparrow$BP, $\downarrow$HDL cholesterol) but improving triglycerides. There is no evidence yet that intensified control of itself confers macrovascular advantage over other treatments, but a specific study is in progress (VADT, USA).

It is widely believed that if insulin treatment is intensive enough, good glycaemic control can always be achieved, and statements like 'the potential for glucose lowering with insulin is unlimited' are found throughout the literature. In real life, however, this is not the case. A substantial proportion of patients taking large doses of insulin (>100 U/day) have very poor glycaemic control (HbA$_{1c}$ >9–10%) a few years after starting insulin, as predicted from the UKPDS; clinically a particularly notable group in the UK is older South Asian women with ischaemic heart disease, who appear to be exceptionally insulin resistant. Most, but not all, of these patients were obese or very obese when they started insulin. However, the converse also occurs: some very overweight patients remain in stable and satisfactory glycaemic control on what appears to be very small doses of insulin. This variability of response, which is not evident from RCT data in large study populations, must be recognised, and should be discussed with patients.

The practical problem therefore is that, like triple oral therapy, it is not possible to predict which overweight individuals will respond well to insulin. Given the difficulty of withdrawing insulin treatment once it has been started, a useful pragmatic approach is therefore to give patients a trial of triple oral therapy for about 4 months to assess response before starting insulin. In RCTs, short-term (up to 6 months) improvements in glycaemic control are similar with insulin and triple oral therapy, and weight gain is also similar. Pioglitazone over 3 years, as reported in the PROACTIVE study, significantly reduced progression to insulin treatment, while maintaining stable glycaemic control. All these considerations suggest more prominence should be given to glitazones in these complex patients.

Initiating insulin treatment

Many insulin regimens are in use:

- basal (overnight) isophane or glargine at bedtime + OHAs
- premixed (30/70) insulin with the evening meal + OHAs
- twice-daily premixed insulin with metformin but without sulphonylurea
- basal-bolus regimen with metformin but without sulphonylurea.

Minor differences in glycaemic outcome are described, but they are likely to be of little or no clinical significance. Early studies used lente or ultralente insulins, but these are now obsolete.

Basal (overnight) insulin + daytime OHAs

This is probably the best starting regimen. Isophane or long-acting analogue insulin, usually given at night, is as effective as twice-daily premixed insulin or basal-bolus insulin, at least in the medium term. It causes less hypoglycaemia, less weight gain, and is more acceptable to these patients who have feared insulin treatment for many years.

OHAs should be left at their current doses (but sulphonylurea and metformin reduced to maximum effective doses – see above for sulphonylurea doses; metformin maintained at 2 g daily, or maximum tolerated). One study suggested that maintaining sulphonylurea + metformin was less effective than metformin alone. Either approach is reasonable.

Isophane insulin should be started at bedtime, e.g. Humulin I or Insulatard at a dose equivalent to usual fasting levels (therefore usually 8–14 U). The smoother action of glargine causes slightly less nocturnal hypoglycaemia, but there appears to be no difference in final HbA_{1c} levels, and isophane insulin is still the most commonly used basal insulin in type 2 diabetes.

Dose titration

These patients have been in poor glycaemic control for many months or years, so there is no need for rapid dose titration (as in type 1 diabetes, rapid dose titration, causing an initial rapid fall in HbA_{1c}, may risk temporary exacerbation of retinopathy). Either a fixed absolute rate of increase, e.g. 4 units every week, or a 10% increase every week, is appropriate. Self-adjustment of the dose with a written regimen, targeting FBG <6 mmol/L, is the most effective approach. An average daily dose of 60–65 U in the VA CSDM feasibility study, now a decade old, maintained reasonable glycaemic control (HbA_{1c} 7.4–7.6%) over 2 years. Even when basal-bolus regimens are used, ~70% of the improvement in glycaemic control is attributable to the basal insulin. Patients should know that whatever regimen is used, they are likely to require a final dose of 40–80 U; many believe that a final dose of more than 20 U is very high, and this is true in comparison with some type 1 patients, and in comparison with their starting doses.

The advantages of this regimen are:

- ease of implementation, and highly acceptable to patients
- low incidence of hypoglycaemia
- can be adapted to a basal-bolus regimen as required
- isophane or long-acting analogue insulin can be given as effectively in the morning as at bedtime; this is particularly valuable in:
  - the occasional patient with good fasting glucose levels
  - the elderly receiving insulin from district nursing services. Because of the slow onset of action of isophane, breakfast can be taken at the usual time, and insulin given before or up to 1 hour after breakfast (isophane onset of action at about 2 hours). Long-acting analogues may be especially safe in this situation.

The disadvantages are:

- still slightly unfamiliar. Patients sometimes want to move to insulin-alone regimens, without the complexity of additional OHAs
- increased side-effects with multiple agents
- possibly lower compliance with a complex regimen.

Other regimens

The most convenient is twice-daily fixed mixture starting at a low dose, e.g. 12 U with breakfast, 8 U with the evening meal. Mixtures containing soluble analogues are more convenient, as they can be given with, during, or after a meal, but there is no convincing evidence for glycaemic superiority compared with standard soluble/isophane mixtures. Continue metformin, and some also continue a long-acting sulphonylurea, e.g.

glimepiride, though the benefit of a sulphonylurea in these patients with long-standing diabetes and β-cell depletion is probably small. RCTs usually use rapid dose titration, but again there is no compelling need to increase each dose by more than 4 U each week in these patients with long-standing poor glycaemic control, and slow titration may reduce the risk of hypoglycaemia. Consider moving to a basal-bolus regimen in the same way as in type 1 diabetes (see Chapter 5) in patients poorly controlled on twice-daily mixtures at total daily doses >~70 U. However, this should be done with caution and humility; the additional benefit in many patients may be small, and there is no virtue in persisting with multiple-dose insulin regimens when glycaemic control (and often weight as well) is not improving, or even worsening.

Management of type 2 patients poorly controlled on insulin

One of the most difficult problems in diabetes management, characterised by:

- glycaemic control that has not improved since starting insulin, or improved transiently but has returned to pre-insulin-treatment levels – or worse
- high daily insulin doses, often >1 U/kg body weight, or >100 U, frequently in a twice-daily fixed mixture or basal-bolus regimen
- increasing weight, with associated worsening insulin resistance features (↑BP, deteriorating lipid profile).

There are no simple explanations or easy solutions, other than recognising that insulin treatment (alone or in combination with currently available OHAs) is an imperfect treatment for type 2 diabetes. However, the following could be attempted:

- adding metformin up to 1 g b.d. The results are variable, but trials show a fall in fasting glucose levels of 2–5 mmol/L, HbA_{1c} up to 1%.
- if HbA_{1c} is not too high, e.g. around 8%, trying very slowly to reduce insulin doses with the aim of withdrawing (or at least minimising) it and substituting a full OHA regimen, usually triple oral therapy. A full support package, including comprehensive dietary advice, and careful home blood glucose monitoring, needs to be in place. Glitazones are not currently licensed for use with insulin in the UK, though RCTs have confirmed the safety and utility of the combination

- dealing vigorously with all cardiovascular risk factors. Glycaemic control itself, on current evidence, is a relatively weak risk factor for cardiovascular disease, and dyslipidaemia and hypertension are important risk factors for the progression of microvascular complications as well as macrovascular disease.

New developments

Combined PPARα and γ agonists (glitazars)

Several compounds, for example muraglitazar and tesaglitazar, have been developed that combine the effects of the glitazones with the lipid-modifying properties (especially triglyceride-lowering and HDL-raising) of the fibric acid drugs, which are PPARα agonists. The side-effect profile of the glitazars is similar to that of the glitazones, though fluid retention and heart failure seem to be more frequent.

Gut hormones – incretins

Over the past 40 years a variety of gut hormones that increase β-cell insulin release in response to nutrients, especially glucose, in the upper gastrointestinal tract, have been characterised. The best-known are GIP (glucose-dependent insulinotropic polypeptide) and GLP-1 (glucagon-like polypeptide-1), but only GLP-1 appears to have clinically useful effects. GLP-1 analogues will be introduced shortly into clinical practice. They have several actions that complement those of existing oral hypoglycaemic agents, for example:

- ↓glucagon secretion
- slow gastric emptying
- ↑glucose-dependent insulin secretion
- ↓food intake and weight
- β-cell trophic effect. Demonstrated experimentally and also in some clinical studies.

Depending on baseline glycaemic control they reduce HbA_{1c} by ~0.5–1.0%.

Liraglutide is a long-acting analogue of GLP-1.

Exenatide is a GLP-1 receptor agonist. It combines effectively with metformin. Both liraglutide and exenatide are relatively resistant to degradation by DPP-IV (dipeptidyl peptidase, see below), thereby prolonging their therapeutic effect compared with the very short-lived native peptides. Both require s.c. injection, either once-daily (liraglutide) or b.d. (exenatide), but doses are fixed, so in practice they will be easier to manage than insulin.

Pramlintide, a synthetic analogue of amylin, a hormone co-secreted with insulin from the pancreas, has similar effects as the incretins – but is not itself an incretin, because it is not gut-derived. It is also likely to be introduced soon, also requires twice-daily s.c. injection, and because it does not have a primary pancreatic effect can be used in both type 1 and type 2 patients.

DPP-IV (dipeptidyl peptidase) inhibitors (gliptins) are orally active agents that inhibit the enzyme that naturally breaks down GLP-1, thereby prolonging its effects. Several, e.g. vildagliptin, are in late-stage development.

Because of their unique mode of action, the effect of these agents is likely to be additive to other drugs in use, especially in view of their modest but consistent effects in reducing weight.

Bariatric surgery

Bariatric surgery encompasses all surgical procedures to reduce weight, primarily adjustable gastric banding and gastric bypass, the latter causing greater weight loss. They are increasingly used, though little in the UK, and have dramatic effects on glycaemia even before there has been significant weight loss – changes in gut hormones, including GLP-1, are probably responsible. The beneficial effects on all metabolic aspects of diabetes are sustained in observational studies up to 16 years. NICE suggests considering bariatric surgery in diabetic patients with a BMI of 35–40.

8 INFECTIONS IN DIABETES

Infections in patients with diabetes are a persistent trap for both the inexperienced and world-wise diabetes physician. High blood glucose levels predispose to some acute infections, especially postoperative, but multiple mechanisms are involved, especially the effects of long-standing hyperglycaemia on small and large blood vessels, and the nervous and immune systems. Only candidal and staphylococcal infections of the skin and mucosae appear to be 'specific' to poorly controlled patients (Fig. 8.1). Continual vigilance is required: whenever an unwell diabetic patient presents, the possibility of infection should be considered.

There are countless case reports of unusual infections in diabetes, but few well-conducted prospective studies or RCTs. While there is a reasonable evidence base for treatment of diabetic foot infections, infections elsewhere remain a real diagnostic and treatment challenge.

Types of infections

- Common infections are also common in diabetes – though there is still controversy whether or not chest or urinary tract infections are in fact more common in people with well-controlled diabetes.
- Common infections occurring in unusual sites (especially staphylococcal infections, see below).
- Common infections giving rise to atypical clinical pictures (e.g. intra-abdominal sepsis).
- Unusual infections occurring in unusual sites. Some serious infections appear to be relatively specific to diabetes (e.g. rhinocerebral mucormycosis, 'malignant' otitis externa, Fournier's gangrene); the whole urinary tract and the limbs appear to be susceptible to invasive gas-forming organisms.

Chest infections

Advanced autonomic neuropathy may impair the perception of pleuritic pain, and there may be some impairment of sensation of dyspnoea. Several studies have found that the risk of death in community-acquired pneumonia in diabetic patients was no greater than in non-diabetic subjects, but there is a concern that these studies may conceal

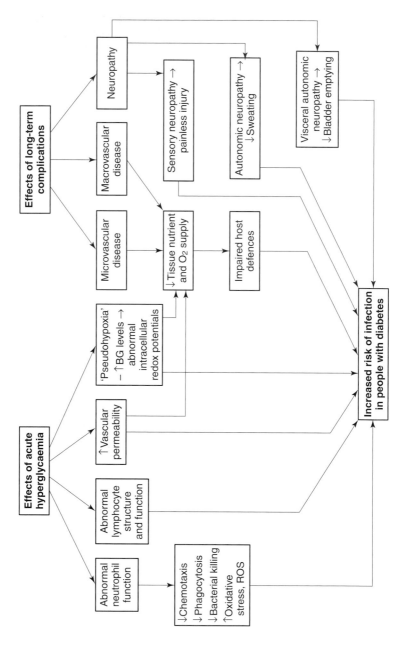

Figure 8.1 Factors leading to increased risk of infection in people with diabetes. ROS, reactive oxygen species.

a greater out-of-hospital mortality. Pneumococcal and influenzal infections do not seem to be more common, but are associated with increased morbidity and mortality, highlighting the need for widespread immunisation in diabetic patients.

Infections with certain organisms are more common in diabetes:

- *Staphylococcus aureus*
- *Mycobacterium tuberculosis*
- Gram-negative organisms, especially *Klebsiella pneumoniae*, which is especially associated with empyema.

Infections after CABG

Diabetes is consistently identified as a powerful predictor of major superficial and deep infections (including mediastinitis, thoracotomy site, septicaemia, vein harvest site) after coronary bypass graft surgery. Renal failure and obesity (BMI 30–40) carry a similar level of risk.

Urinary tract infections (UTI)

Contributory factors are not well understood, but there is general agreement that bladder dysfunction resulting from neuropathy is a major factor.

Asymptomatic bacteriuria

There is no difference between diabetic and non-diabetic men, but it is twice as common in diabetic women as non-diabetic women. Asymptomatic bacteriuria detected in routine screening should probably not be treated: a study in 2002 found that after initial treatment of asymptomatic bacteriuria, there was no difference in the rate of development of subsequent definite UTI. This finding has recently been challenged, and vigilance is required when for any reason urine cultures are found to be positive.

Symptomatic UTI

The upper urinary tract is involved in ~80% of UTI in diabetic patients, and more commonly bilaterally. Other complications are more common.

Table 8.1 Urinary tract infections in diabetes

Infection	Clinical features	Diagnostic procedures	Microbiology	Comments
Cystitis	Frequency, dysuria, suprapubic pain	Urine culture. USS renal tract to exclude upper tract involvement	*Escherichia coli*, *Proteus* spp.	Less common organisms include *Klebsiella* spp., Group B streptococci, enterococci, *Pseudomonas*
Pyelonephritis	Fever, loin pain	Urine culture, USS renal tract	*E. coli*, *Proteus* spp.	Consider bilateral involvement
Emphysematous pyelonephritis	Fever, loin pain, poor response to antibotics	Plain x-ray, USS, CT scan	*E. coli*, other Gram-negative bacilli	ITU, emergency nephrectomy often needed, hyperbaric oxygen may help
Perinephric abscess	Fever, loin pain, poor response to antibiotics (fever persisting for more than 4 days after start of antibiotic treatment)	USS, CT scan	*E. coli*, other Gram-negative bacilli, *Staph. aureus* from haematogenous spread	Consider surgical drainage
Papillary necrosis	Fever, loin and abdominal pain	May be found on USS, IVU		
Fungal	All the above can occur, depending on site of infection	Difficult to diagnose, especially difficult to distinguish from colonisation; urine culture	*Candida* spp.	Oral fluconazole

Modified from Joshi N *et al.* Infections in patients with diabetes mellitus. *NEJM*, 1999; 341: 1906–12. ITU, intensive therapy unit; IVU, intravascular ultrasound; USS, ultrasound scan.

Management

Treat pyelonephritis in the same way as non-diabetic patients, but always admit for i.v. antibiotics and to intensify diabetes treatment. There is also likely to be associated decreased appetite and nausea and vomiting, and a risk of DKA/HHS. Bacterial cystitis should be treated for at least 7 days, possibly 14 days, longer than in a non-diabetic patient because of the tendency to involve the upper urinary tract.

Always be vigilant for the development of perinephric abscess and the rare but frequently fatal emphysematous pyelonephritis.

Choice of antibiotic

Either i.v. co-amoxiclav 0.6–1.2 g t.d.s., or in the penicillin sensitive patient, a fluoroquinolone, either ciprofloxacin 500 mg b.d. or levofloxacin 500 mg o.d. should be the first choice. In the very ill patient, use ceftazidime 0.5–1 g 12-hourly, or cefuroxime 0.75–1.5 g 6–8 hourly.

Gentamicin remains valuable in sick patients. Do not use if serum creatinine >300 µmol/L. Once-daily dosing is appropriate in patients with normal renal function (serum creatinine <120 µmol/L), starting at 5 mg/kg to a maximum of 400 mg. Even in normal renal function, trough levels should be monitored at least every 3 days (<1 mg/L).

Once fever and systemic symptoms have settled, transfer to oral antibiotics and maintain for 14 days.

Recurrent UTIs require ultrasound of the urinary tract and involvement of the urologists, but low-dose prophylaxis can be given with daily cefalexin or ciprofloxacin 250 mg or trimethoprim 100 mg.

Abdominal infections

As with all infections in diabetes, vigilance is mandatory as signs and symptoms may be subtle.

The more common specific abdominal infection is peritonitis in patients on peritoneal dialysis. It is usually caused by Gram-positive organisms, predominantly *Staph. aureus*, but Gram-negative infections occur – those caused by *Pseudomonas* and *Serratia marcescens* have a poorer outlook.

Other reported infections include:

- emphysematous cholecystitis; usually polymicrobial – Gram-negative + anaerobes

- gynaecological infections – occult pelvic abscess should always be considered
- hepatic abscess (most commonly *Klebsiella*) – uncommon in UK practice
- retroperitoneal abscesses.

Soft tissue infections

Cellulitis

A spreading infection of the epidermis, dermis and subcutaneous fat. It is common in diabetes and, in the presence of chronic leg oedema, sometimes difficult to treat.

Without coexisting foot ulceration (but always check carefully for minor skin breaks and interdigital fungal infections), treat as in a person without diabetes, covering the most likely organisms, i.e. *Staph. aureus* and β-haemolytic streptococci, usually group A (*Streptococcus pyogenes*). Blood cultures are usually negative, but if there is blistering, the fluid should be cultured from an unruptured blister. Exclude deep venous thrombosis.

Oral antibiotics are suitable if the legs are not involved, or there is very local involvement of the legs, but err on the side of caution, and 24–48 hours of i.v. antibiotics (ambulatory setting where possible) is preferable. In the penicillin-tolerant patient, high dose co-amoxiclav (e.g. 1.2 g t.d.s) is appropriate, and has a wider spectrum than the commonly used benzylpenicillin + flucloxacillin. Antibiotics that might be less effective, e.g. macrolides (erythromycin, clarithromycin), flucloxacillin alone (which is not effective against streptococci) or metronidazole (anaerobes are not usually involved unless there is abscess formation) should be avoided. Observe the response; laboratory measurements (CRP, WBC) can improve before the clinical state. The antibiotic regimen should be modified if necessary – strengthening the anti-Gram-positive regimen (e.g. adding benzylpenicillin or clindamycin) is often effective. Resistant cases, particularly where there is a large volume of infected soft tissue with oedema, can take 2 or more weeks of in-patient antibiotic treatment. Widespread desquamation on recovery is characteristic of streptococcal infections.

Diabetic foot ulceration (see also Chapter 11)

The choice of antibiotic is difficult, because several factors have to be taken into account:

- chronicity
- depth: superficial, deep, bone involvement
- where the infection was acquired: community or hospital, and associated likelihood of particular organisms, e.g. MRSA in frequently hospitalised patients, presence of sensitive streptococci in community-acquired infection, mixed growths in chronic infection, presence of anaerobic/gas-forming organisms
- presence of ischaemia and osteomyelitis.

Deep cultures, especially of tissue, are important, but results are unlikely to be available for several days. The broadest possible spectrum is required in most instances, but *Staph. aureus* and streptococci should always be covered.

There are no established guidelines for antibiotic treatment of an infected diabetic foot ulcer, but consider the following points:

- Because signs of infection are often attenuated or obscured in diabetic neuropathy, the patient should never be under-treated; it is always better to err on the side of caution, and admit for i.v. treatment if in doubt, especially if there is associated cellulitis or purulent exudate. Abscesses are often difficult to detect clinically in oedematous feet, and may become apparent only when surgical or podiatrist debridement has been carried out. Infections in the ulcerated foot can spread with alarming speed.
- The traditional trio of antibiotics has been benzylpenicillin, flucloxacillin and metronidazole, but high-dose co-amoxiclav or ciprofloxacin/levofloxacin in the penicillin-allergic patient is probably the best initial option unless there is severe spreading infection, in which case ceftriaxone/ceftazidime will give broader cover, with some anti-staphylococcal reinforcement, e.g. clindamycin.
- Liaise with the surgical team over management, and with the microbiologists about antibiotic treatment in difficult cases. Abscesses, not uncommon, need surgical drainage.

Osteomyelitis

Radiologically, osteomyelitis is often difficult to diagnose, especially in distal phalanges. Osteomyelitis in the foot usually occurs adjacent to an ulcer – in the diabetic foot, osteomyelitis 'never' occurs in the presence of completely healed skin, though small puncture wounds, especially in flexures of the toes, can sometimes heal up having allowed infection

101

Table 8.2 Antibiotics frequently used in diabetic foot infections, and their spectrum of activity

Antibiotic	Formulation		Relative activity against specific pathogens				Comments
	Oral	i.v./i.m.	S. aureus	Strepto-cocci	Entero-bacteriaceae	Anaer-obes	
Penicillins							
Benzylpenicillin		Yes	+	++++	+	++	Penicillin V should not be used
Flucloxacillin	Yes	Yes	++++	+++	0	++	Relatively poorly tolerated, especially in high doses; delayed cholestatic jaundice can occur. Avoid long courses
Co-amoxiclav	Yes	Yes	++++	++++	++	+++	Important broad spectrum agent; also associated with cholestatic jaundice, especially in the over 65s
Amoxicillin/ampicillin	Yes	Yes	+	++++	++	++	Co-amoxiclav preferable
Piperacillin/tazobactam	No	Yes	++++	++++	+++	++++	Very broad spectrum, including *Pseudomonas*
Cephalosporins							
Cefuroxime	No	Yes	++++	++++	++	++	

							Comments
Ceftriaxone/ceftazidime	No	Yes	+++	+++	++++	++	Useful agent in severe infections in penicillin-sensitive patients
Fluroquinolones							
Ciprofloxacin	Yes	Yes	+++	++	++++	0	Good bone penetration; well tolerated in long courses
Levofloxacin	Yes	Yes	+++	+++	++++	+	
Anaerobic agents							
Clindamycin	Yes	Yes	++++	+++	0	++++	Good bone penetration; important anti-staphylococcal agent. Diarrhoea and antibiotic-associated colitis recognised side-effects
Metronidazole	Yes	0	0	0	0	++++	
Others							
Vancomycin/teicoplanin	No	Yes	++++	+++	0	++	For MRSA
Imipenem–cilastatin	No	Yes	++++	++++	++++	+++	Similar spectrum to piperacillin/tazobactam
Rifampicin	Yes	No	++++	0	+++	++++	In combination anti-staphylococcal regimen

After Lipsky BA and Berendt AR. *Diab Met Res Rev*, 2000; 16 (Suppl 1): S42–46.

to enter. If there are appearances suggesting osteomyelitis with no clinical ulceration, then consider Charcot neuroarthropathy (see Chapter 11).

Osteomyelitis may progress rapidly; always compare with previous films. If osteomyelitis is suspected, then repeat films every month to detect subtle cortical changes.

The gold standard investigation, where clinical suspicion is high, is MRI, where oedema in the bone may be apparent. However, MRI will not reliably distinguish between osteomyelitis and early Charcot neuroarthropathy.

Osteomyelitis is almost always caused by *Staph. aureus*. Open biopsy and culture is needed for definite confirmation, but this is rarely needed except when there is high suspicion of another organism, or failure to respond to prolonged high-dose anti-staphylococcal antibiotics.

Necrotising fasciitis

Fulminating gangrene of skin and subcutaneous fat and dermis with a high mortality (~30%). The gangrene is caused by thrombosis in the subcutaneous vasculature. Cutaneous signs initially may not be very impressive, though irregular dusky blue and black patches with bullae appear within a few days. Septicaemia with multiorgan failure can be fulminant. Always think about it in diabetic patients with cellulitis; culture widely and check CK. Necrotising fasciitis is a surgical emergency.

Microbiology
- Predominantly Lancefield group A β-haemolytic streptococci (*Strep. pyogenes*).
- Less severe infections are seen with group C and G β-haemolytic streptococci; diabetes is a definite risk factor.
- Fournier's gangrene (genital necrotising fasciitis): *Staph. aureus, E. coli*, anaerobes (clostridia, bacteroides, or anaerobic streptococci).
- *Vibrio vulnificus* is increasingly described, found in southern hemisphere warm coastal waters.

Management
Intensive supporting therapy is needed for shock, together with immediate surgical advice regarding degree of debridement/amputation.

Antibiotics, high-dose i.v. benzylpenicillin (e.g. >14 g/day) and clindamycin (900 mg t.d.s.) should be given for suspected *Strep. pyogenes* infection; metronidazole + cephalosporin if Fournier's gangrene is suspected. Where available, hyperbaric oxygen therapy is probably beneficial.

Uncommon infections characteristic of diabetes

'Malignant' otitis externa

'Malignant' otitis externa is usually caused by *Pseudomonas aeruginosa*. Disproportionate pain, discharge and hearing loss are the warning features, but diagnosis is often delayed. Involvement of the skull itself (osteomyelitis) with secondary cerebral venous thrombosis are late manifestations. Joint surgical management with the ENT team and prolonged (6 weeks) systemic and topical anti-pseudomonal antibiotics are needed.

Rhinocerebral mucormycosis

This is extremely uncommon, and said to be associated with diabetic ketoacidosis. It starts with face or eye pain, with progressive ocular involvement – proptosis, ophthalmoplegia, with severe constitutional upset. Cavernous sinus thrombosis, and jugular vein or carotid artery thrombosis are described. MRI, prompt involvement of the ENT and microbiology teams, and prolonged treatment with antifungal agents are required.

Ophthalmic infections

Staphylococcal endophthalmitis after cataract surgery, though rare, is more common in diabetes. There are also sporadic reports of endogenous endophthalmitis resulting from septicaemia originating from an infection elsewhere, especially diabetic foot lesions (*Staphylococcus*), liver abscesses (*Klebsiella*) and urinary tract infection (*E. coli*). A potentially serious eye infection should always be considered when a diabetic patient presents with a red eye.

Musculoskeletal infections

Multiple varieties have been described, including:

- epidural abscess
- discitis
- psoas abscess
- vertebral osteomyelitis.

Staphylococcus is the predominating organism, but *Streptococcus* and *Pneumococcus* are also found. These are often indolent infections that are difficult to diagnose; they should be considered in poorly controlled, complicated diabetic patients with focal spinal pain. Isotope bone scan and MRI are needed, with expert microbiological and neurosurgical/orthopaedic help.

9 DIABETIC EYE DISEASE

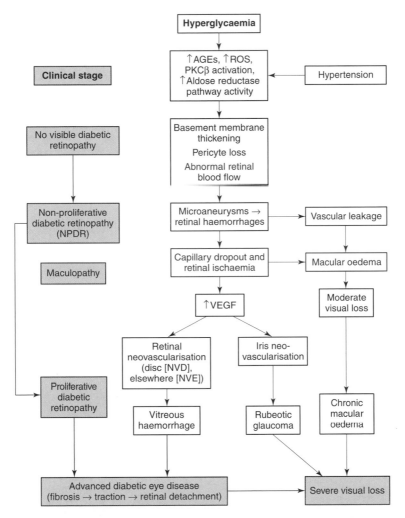

Figure 9.1 Clinicopathological correlations in diabetic retinopathy. AGE, advanced glycation end products; PKCβ, protein kinase C β isoform; ROS, reaction oxygen species; VEGF vascular endothelial growth factor.

Diabetic retinopathy is the most common clinically significant microvascular complication of diabetes, but cataract is the most common ocular complication (prevalence ~60% in the age group 30–54 years). Raised intraocular pressure and chronic open angle glaucoma are also probably associated with diabetes, and retinal venous and arterial occlusions are also more common. Eye screening in diabetes should therefore include all these important pathologies – and of course refractive errors are common as well.

Retinopathy is uncommon in the first 5 years of type 1 diabetes, but certainly occurs, and may become more common as atypical slow-onset forms of type 1 diabetes emerge. Studies from the 1980s show a near-100% prevalence of some degree of retinopathy after 15–20 years of type 1 diabetes, about 50% having proliferative changes. This is not the case today: perhaps up to 20% of type 1 diabetic patients will be completely free of retinopathy after 15 years – and many of these will also have no evidence of other microvascular complications. Several recent studies show decreasing rates of advanced diabetic retinopathy and blindness in type 1 diabetes, but 30% still have proliferative retinopathy after 10 years.

The picture is different in type 2 diabetes, where 20–30% have retinopathy at diagnosis, and 10–25% have proliferative retinopathy 10 years after diagnosis. As in nephropathy, therefore, the burden of retinopathy work for ophthalmology departments comes from type 2 patients.

Screening for diabetic retinopathy

The recommendation is still that all adult patients should be screened annually for diabetic retinopathy. There is sound evidence that in patients with no evidence of retinopathy the screening interval could be increased to 18 months or even 2 years, but this selective approach is too complex to implement at present. Major changes in screening protocols have occurred in the past 5 years; the National Service Framework for diabetes (2002) has suggested digital camera retinal screening as the optimum method, but secure systems using community optometrists are in place in many areas. Ophthalmologists are now doing less of this work, and, importantly, very little screening occurs in the diabetes clinic – a major change from the situation 10 years ago. There is therefore much less need for the general diabetologist to be able to screen for retinopathy, but it is a skill that is still required. Some patients evade the community screening programmes, and cannot be relied on to get back into the system once they are discharged from hospital. Direct ophthalmoscopy is therefore an important part of in-patient screening of newly diagnosed and poorly controlled patients. More importantly from the generalist point of view, retinopathy of any degree should stimulate close scrutiny for associated microvascular complications, and control of risk factors for its progression.

Risk factors for progression of background retinopathy

- Unsurprising: diabetes duration, glycaemic control (especially associated with proliferative retinopathy), systolic blood pressure (associated with maculopathy).
- Dyslipidaemia has been identified in some studies, including type 1 patients – especially elevated triglycerides and low HDL cholesterol. This has been expanded in some studies to suggest that the metabolic syndrome itself is associated with risk of progression.

Examination

Visual acuity

The eyes should be tested separately with glasses, if worn, using a standard Snellen test chart for distance. If vision is not normal (acuity 6/6 or 6/9), the eyes should be tested with a pin-hole. Acuity will improve where there is a refractive error or early cataract, but will not improve if there is macular disease or more advanced cataract.

Background retinopathy usually has no effect on visual acuity, and unless there is macular involvement, even severe pre-proliferative and proliferative retinopathy is associated with normal visual acuity. Onset of macular oedema is characteristically associated with a marked decrease in visual acuity.

Pupil dilatation

- Must be done properly in order to perform a proper retinal examination. It may be possible to get a good view of the retina in a young person examined in a darkened room without dilatation – but it is best to get into the habit of dilating.
- Warn the patient that the drops will sting.

- Check that the eye drops are correct and in date.
- Instil one drop of 1% tropicamide in the lower conjunctival sac of each eye; do not place on the cornea.
- Patients with dark irises often dilate poorly with tropicamide. Consider using, in addition, one drop of 2.5% phenylephrine. The combination is often used routinely in ophthalmology clinics.
- Dilatation is complete in about 15 minutes.
- Tropicamide does not significantly impair accommodation and patients with normal visual acuity can drive afterwards. 'Reversing' dilatation with pilocarpine is not usually done, as the effect of tropicamide lasts only 1-2 hours.
- The risk of precipitating acute angle closure glaucoma is vanishingly small, but do not dilate pupils in patients with known glaucoma.
- Previous intraocular surgery is also a contraindication to dilatation, but the presence of successful lens implants is not.

Red reflex and examination of anterior structures
- Use a fully charged ophthalmoscope.
- Use a +10 lens.
- Hold the ophthalmoscope 20–25 cm from the eye.
- Illuminate the red reflex.
- Move the ophthalmoscope towards the eye until the anterior structures are visible.
- Lens opacities appear black; if the central red reflex is present, then the cataract is not obstructing the visual axis.

Examination of the retina
- Gradually decrease the number on the ophthalmoscope until the retinal vessels come into focus.
- Leave the examination of the macula to the end, as examination causes marked pupillary constriction.
- Start with the optic disc: examine for cupping, pallor, and disc defect.
- Examine each quadrant separately, following the major vessels. Look for hypertensive as well as diabetic changes: arteriovenous nipping is easiest to find in the upper outer quadrant, where there is the greatest number of arteriovenous crossings.
- Finally, examine the area temporal to the macula, and then the macula itself.

- Do not spend too long examining the fundi (maximum ~2 min each eye) or you will start detecting retinopathy that does not exist.

Classification of retinopathy

An international retinopathy severity scale has recently been proposed, based on the presence of red lesions only (Table 9.1). This scheme abolishes the categories of background and pre-proliferative retinopathy, is simple, and is likely to become widely used. The notes below use the current classification.

Table 9.1 Proposed classification of retinopathy

Proposed disease severity level	Findings on dilated ophthalmoscopy
No apparent retinopathy	No abnormalities
Mild NPDR	Microaneurysms only
Moderate NPDR	More than just microaneurysms, but less than severe NPDR
Severe NPDR (4:2:1 rule)	Any of the following: • >20 intraretinal haemorrhages in each of 4 quadrants • definite venous beading in 2+ quadrants prominent intraretinal microvascular • abnormalities in 1+ quadrant but no signs of proliferative retinopathy
PDR	One or more of the following: • neovascularisation • vitreous/preretinal haemorrhage

NPDR, non-proliferative diabetic retinopathy; PDR, proliferative retinopathy.

Non-proliferative retinopathy

Background retinopathy (see Plate 1)

Microaneurysms
Red, intraretinal lesions occur most frequently at the posterior pole of the eye, around the disc and macula. They occur in areas of capillary non-perfusion and show leakage of fluorescein. It is worthwhile trying to estimate the number of microaneurysms, as this has some prognostic significance; the greater the number, the higher the likelihood of progression to proliferative retinopathy.

Hard exudates

Waxy yellow dots or plaques are formed by extravasated plasma proteins. They occur early in diabetic retinopathy, but they are only of visual significance if they form at or near the macula.

Intraretinal haemorrhages (see Plate 2)

There are various types:

- dot and blot
- flame-shaped haemorrhages in the retinal nerve fibre layer (often striated). These are also characteristic of non-diabetic hypertension, and sometimes also transiently occur in people with well-controlled type 1 diabetes
- deeper haemorrhages with irregular outlines
- large, dark, 'cluster' haemorrhages.

Cotton-wool spots (soft exudates)

These are white, fluffy-edged lesions, quite unlike hard exudates, and represent accumulation of axoplasmic material adjacent to a retinal infarct. An occasional cotton-wool spot is of little significance, but in greater numbers (>5) they are thought to indicate:

- rapidly advancing retinopathy
- associated hypertension
- unrelated disease, e.g. vasculitis.

Multiple soft exudates are frequent accompaniments of pre-proliferative retinopathy, though this view has been challenged recently.

Management

No ophthalmological treatment is needed, but it is good practice to repeat fundoscopy every 6 months, especially for patients with poor glycaemic control (e.g. HbA_{1c} ≥9%) if there are multiple lesions of background retinopathy, as there is a risk of rapid progression. The presence of background changes, while of no interest to the ophthalmologist, should remind the diabetes team that all risk factors for progression (see above) should be addressed vigorously. There is good evidence from the DCCT that HbA_{1c} sustained at <7.0% for several years is likely to lead to regression of early changes in type 1 diabetes. Intensive glucose control in the UKPDS also reduced the risk of progression of retinopathy by about 20% in type 2 diabetes.

Several studies have shown that transient worsening of retinopathy, sometimes dramatic, can occur with very rapid tightening of glycaemic control in both type 1 and type 2 diabetes, even when there are only minor pre-existing degrees of retinopathy. Vigilance, therefore, is especially important in the following groups of patients:

- type 1 patients during the pre-conception and early pregnancy periods
- patients starting CSII
- thin, insulin-deficient type 2 patients, with very poor control (e.g. HbA_{1c} >12%) who may have a very dramatic response to insulin therapy
- any patient with known retinopathy in whom a rapid fall in HbA_{1c} has occurred – for whatever reason.

Blood pressure treatment

Intensive BP control reduces the risk of progression of retinopathy in both type 1 and 2 diabetes. Prospective studies have not been able to identify any antihypertensive agents with benefit beyond their BP lowering effect, but the EUCLID/EURODIAB study (1998) suggested that ACE inhibitor treatment with lisinopril was associated with a decreased risk of retinopathy progression, and progression to proliferative retinopathy in type 1 patients. More conclusive guidance may result from the DIRECT study, not yet reported, using the angiotensin receptor blocker (ARB) candesartan. Many patients with retinopathy will already be taking angiotensin blocking treatment for hypertension or microalbuminuria. The evidence, however, is not yet compelling enough to warrant treatment with angiotensin blockade in normotensive type 1 patients with isolated background retinopathy and no microalbuminuria.

Pre-proliferative retinopathy

Features that carry increased risk of proliferation, significant risk of sight-threatening retinopathy developing within a year and which must be assessed promptly by an ophthalmologist, comprise:

- venous beading, looping or reduplication
- multiple (>5) cotton-wool spots
- multiple haemorrhages
- intraretinal microvascular abnormalities (IRMAs): vessels that look like new vessels, and which branch abnormally (in frequency,

113

number and angulation). However, unlike new vessels, they are intraretinal and do not lead to preretinal or vitreous haemorrhage. Clinically they are very difficult to spot by the non-expert.

Treatment is with panretinal (scatter) laser photocoagulation, which reduces the risk of severe visual loss by about 50%. However, this is destructive treatment, and frequently leads to loss of peripheral and night vision. Laser treatment is intended to stabilise visual loss, not improve it. Treatment is time-consuming and uncomfortable (blurred vision and pain are common after treatment), and sympathetic discussion is needed to maximise cooperation. Many patients will never have seen a picture of the retina, and photographs are helpful in discussion. The presence of other microvascular complications, especially microalbuminuria/proteinuria, and hypertension should be evaluated. All risk factors (above) must be treated with great vigour.

Proliferative retinopathy (see Plates 3 and 4)

Retinal neovascularisation

This comprises NVE (new vessels elsewhere), arising from veins, usually at a bifurcation; and NVD (disc neovascularisation). Although proliferative retinopathy is characteristic of type 1 diabetes, it frequently occurs in type 2, just as maculopathy is not restricted to type 2 diabetes.

Growth factors, especially vascular endothelial growth factor (VEGF), released from ischaemic retina, lead to proliferation. Proliferating vessels lie in the preretinal space, between the retina and the posterior surface of the vitreous gel, and may bleed into the pre-retinal space or the vitreous (vitreous haemorrhage). Traction retinal detachment occurs through contraction of fibrous tissue associated with the new vessels.

Pre-proliferative changes associated with ischaemia are frequently present.

Treatment

Treatment is by panretinal laser photocoagulation, as above.

Maculopathy (see Plate 5)

Maculopathy is defined as background diabetic retinopathy within 2 disc diameters of the centre of the fovea. It is the more common form of

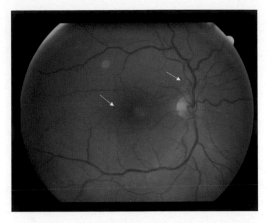

Plate 1 Minor background diabetic retinopathy in long-standing type 1 diabetes, with a few dot and small blot haemorrhages. Of no visual significance, but suggests suboptimal glycaemic control. Though this 'minimal' retinopathy in practice appears to come and go, and is not likely to progress rapidly, it requires strict annual review, preferably with retinal photography, for comparison.

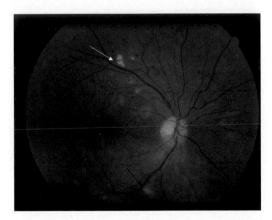

Plate 2 Moderately severe background retinopathy with multiple dot and blot haemorrhages. There are some photographic artefacts in the lower part (black arrow), that can easily mimic true cotton-wool spots (white arrow). Although there are no formal high-risk features here, this degree of retinopathy must be watched carefully, and all risk factors addressed.

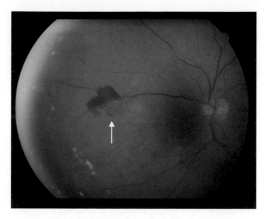

Plate 3 Proliferative diabetic retinopathy: new vessels elsewhere (NVE) – an extensive tuft of new vessels (arrow). There has been a large haemorrhage associated with the abnormal vessels, but at this stage the visual acuity is normal (macula not involved). Unusually, there is little background retinopathy in this view.

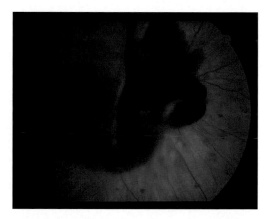

Plate 4 Advanced diabetic retinopathy: type 2 patient, aged 50, with neuropathic foot ulceration and proteinuria. Massive haemorrhages with fluid levels, from proliferative retinopathy (obscured by haemorrhages). This will inevitably be associated with severe, usually rapid onset visual loss. About 8 years after this photograph, the patient is registered partially sighted, has needed several minor toe amputations, but with good podiatric care and footwear is still mobile and independent.

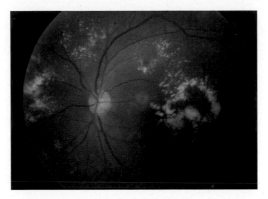

Plate 5 'Classical' extensive maculopathy, with circinate plaques of exudate near the macula and elsewhere, in an African-Caribbean patient with 15 years of type 2 diabetes. The macular oedema, which can be inferred from the circinate exudates, is difficult to treat, and is usually associated with significant visual loss. There is anecdotal evidence that vigorous lowering of LDL levels may help regression of the exudates, but there is usually associated poor glycaemic control and hypertension, all of which should be targeted.

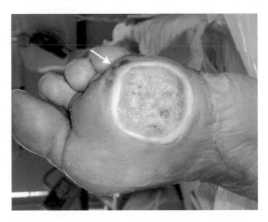

Plate 6 Male, aged 63, long-standing (>20 years) type 2 diabetes. Previous fifth toe amputation, typical, but large, neuropathic ulceration at point of greatest pressure in deformed foot. Note (1) thick callus surrounding the ulcer, which builds up quickly and requires frequent removal; (2) thick adherent exudate on the ulcer base, which must also be removed, usually by scalpel (but larval therapy is sometimes helpful); and (3) areas of haemorrhage into the callus (arrowed). Non-weight-bearing is critical for healing, either bed rest or total contact casting.

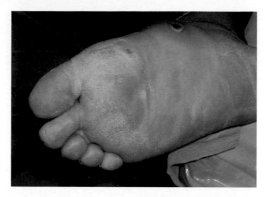

Plate 7 Male, aged 36. Type 1 diabetes, duration 15 years. Rapidly progressing Charcot neuroarthropathy. Previous contralateral below-knee amputation. Heavy alcohol intake. Very short history: twisted ankle and had not recognised that there was an acute problem so had continued to walk on it for 2 weeks. Note the loss of the foot arches, associated with collapse of the mid-foot with medial bony protuberance which has ulcerated. Immobilisation with total contact casting, bisphosphonate treatment and meticulous construction of custom footwear are required.

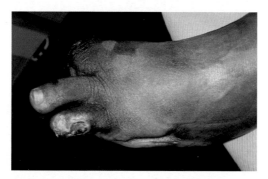

Plate 8 Female, 37 years old, type 1 diabetes, duration 25 years. Haemodialysis for past 5 years. A sadly typical picture of a renal failure patient, with combined advanced neuropathy and ischaemia, and several minor amputations, cumulatively over 4 years, resulting in a foot with little useful function. Note ischaemic third toe with superficial ulceration. Surgical scar from amputation of fourth/fifth digits. Neuroischaemic lesion of the medial side of great toe was caused by exposure to heating system in hospital transport vehicle. The lesion of the third toe is typical of ischaemia resulting from poorly fitting footwear (not the typical plantar ulceration caused by neuropathy).

sight-threatening retinopathy in type 2 diabetes, and visual impairment occurs through macular oedema, macular ischaemia, or most commonly, a combination of the two. Neither can be diagnosed with direct ophthalmoscopy, and though the presence of oedema can be inferred from the frequent finding of a grey patch of retina with central micro-aneurysms and surrounding (circinate) exudates, macular ischaemia can only be diagnosed with fluorescein angiography.

Ophthalmologists use the term 'clinically significant macular oedema' (CSMO) to describe patterns of macular oedema that if not laser treated will result in significant visual loss.

Focal maculopathy

Exudates are typically in a circinate (complete or incomplete) arrangement. This responds well to grid laser treatment. When macular oedema is long-standing, there may be large plaques of exudates at the macula (Plate 5). These are untreatable with laser, but there are case reports of resolution with vigorous lipid-lowering treatment.

Diffuse macular oedema

This is indicated by exudates at the edge of the oedema, but less marked in the macular area itself. Laser treatment can help the oedema, but the visual acuity outcomes are usually poor.

Ischaemic maculopathy

This is suggested by cluster haemorrhages and 'whitening' of vessels as they cross areas of non-perfusion. Laser treatment does not help.

Advanced diabetic eye disease

Advanced diabetic eye disease is visual loss due to complications of proliferative retinopathy, caused by a fibrovascular response to retinal ischaemia. Traction from fibrous tissue may lead to:

- traction retinal detachment
- avulsion of retinal blood vessels, causing haemorrhage:
  - preretinal haemorrhage. Boat-shaped with a horizontal fluid blood level; may be precipitated by hypoglycemia or Valsalva manoeuvre. Often form inferotemporal to the optic disc, and may obscure the macula, leading to acute visual loss. Preretinal haemorrhage implies the presence of proliferative changes,

which may be obscured by the haemorrhage. They sometimes regress spontaneously, but if not, vitrectomy, usually with endolaser photocoagulation, is frequently used, and results are impressive and improving

- vitreous haemorrhage. Usually large, dense haemorrhages that obscure most of the retina. Like preretinal haemorrhage, implies bleeding from proliferating vessels
- neovascularisation of the iris (rubeosis iridis), usually in association with widespread retinal ischaemia or tractional retinal detachment, may lead to rubeotic glaucoma when drainage channels for aqueous humour become blocked. Difficult to treat and visual prognosis is poor.

Cataract

Diabetes is a strong risk factor for cataract, and occurs earlier and progresses faster than in the non-diabetic population. Indications for cataract surgery are:

- impairment of vision that reduces quality of life
- suspicion of retinopathy that is obscured by the cataract.

Cataract surgery is more difficult and associated with poorer visual outcomes. There is an increased complication rate in diabetic patients (e.g. rapid progression of retinopathy, posterior capsule opacification, iris neovascularisation, endophthalmitis).

New developments

Several drugs are in development that are likely to retard progression of pre-proliferative retinopathy or maculopathy. The main interest is in maculopathy, where the most promising is ruboxistaurin (LY333531), an orally active protein kinase C β-isoform antagonist in phase 3 trials. Drugs that either bind VEGF, e.g. pegaptanib, or antagonise it, e.g. ranibizumab, are in development. Somatostatin analogues, requiring intermittent subcutaneous injection, some already in use in endocrine disorders, e.g. acromegaly, are likely also to be introduced. Intravitreal glucocorticoids, e.g. triamcinolone, may be of value in macular oedema, but long-term outcome studies have not reported, and there is concern about raised intraocular pressure and cataract formation.

10   DIABETIC RENAL DISEASE

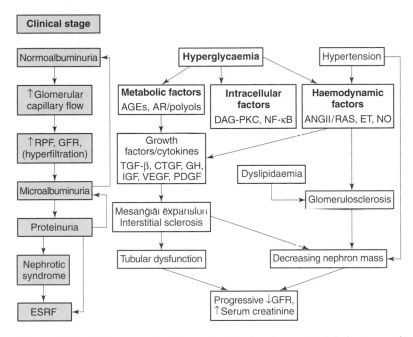

Figure 10.1   Pathogenetic scheme for the development of diabetic renal disease with associated clinical stages (left). AGE, advanced glycation end products; AR, aldose reductase; DAG, diacylglycerol; PKC protein kinase C; NF-κB, nuclear factor; ANGII, angiotensin II, RAS, renin-angiotensin system; ET, endothelin, NO, nitric oxide, TGF, transforming growth factor; CTGF, connective tissue growth factor; VEGF, vascular endothelial growth factor; GH, growth hormone; IGF, insulin-like growth factor; RPF, renal plasma flow; GFR, glomerular filtration rate; ESRF, end-stage renal failure.

Definitions of urinary albumin excretion

These frequently cause confusion. It is important to distinguish the three different measurement methods:

- 24-hour urinary albumin excretion (mg/24 h)
- timed (usually overnight) albumin excretion rate (AER, μg/min)

- spot specimen (usually early morning) expressed as albumin:creatinine ratio (ACR) (mg/mmol, mg/g).

In diabetes practice it is usual to measure urinary **albumin**; once patients transfer to the renal team, the concern is with gram, rather than milligram leakages, and total urinary **protein** is usually measured (urinary albumin $\cong$70% total urinary protein). The distinction is of importance in the microalbuminuric range.

Normoalbuminuria

The normal range of AER is usually quoted as 1.5–20 µg/min, with a geometric mean of 6.5 µg/min $\cong$10 mg/24 h – AER is logarithmically, not normally distributed). This value is similar to the detection limit of most laboratory assays.

Microalbuminuria

- Urinary albumin excretion 30–299 mg/24 h.
- AER 20–199 µg/min.
- ACR ~3–20 mg/mmol.

There may be intermittent stick-positive proteinuria.

Macroalbuminuria

- Urinary albumin excretion $\geq$300 mg/24 h.
- AER $\geq$200 µg/min.
- ACR >20 mg/mmol.

There is invariably persistent 1–3+ stick-positive proteinuria.

Other definitions of macroalbuminuria include urinary **protein** excretion >500 mg/24 h.

Diabetic nephropathy

Diabetic nephropathy is a syndrome comprising:

- macroalbuminuria
- hypertension
- relentlessly deteriorating renal function ($\downarrow$GFR and $\uparrow$serum creatinine).

118

Nephrotic syndrome

There is no formal definition of nephrotic syndrome in terms of albuminuria, but urinary albumin excretion >2.5 g/24 h, that is, more than ~3 g urinary protein excretion/24 h, is often used; the formal triad includes hypoalbuminaemia and an associated dyslipidaemia ($\uparrow$total and LDL cholesterol, to a varying degree, $\uparrow$TG, $\downarrow$HDL cholesterol). Nephrotic syndrome is a high-risk state for rapid deterioration in GFR; is always associated with advanced structural changes on renal biopsy, and is associated with a poor survival (see below). It is not known why certain patients develop the nephrotic syndrome.

Natural history

Successful intervention with antihypertensive agents and angiotensin blockade is now so common that the natural history of the untreated condition is almost only of historical interest. Several long-term longitudinal cohort studies have demonstrated that, like retinopathy, the incidence of diabetic nephropathy in type 1 diabetes is falling, but this may represent just a delay in the peak incidence rate, rather than a true decline.

Type 1 diabetes

Any degree of proteinuria caused by diabetes is unusual in the first 5 years after diagnosis. Microalbuminuria is commonly due to glomerular hyperfiltration secondary to poor glycaemic control – but little is known about the course of this.

In a population of type 1 patients, around 15% will have microalbuminuria, 5% macroalbuminuria, and 3% will be in renal failure. The incidence of microalbuminuria and macroalbuminuria increase at about 2% a year, so that after 25 years, about one-third of patients will have diabetic nephropathy. Pre-pubertal duration of type 1 diabetes may contribute less than post-pubertal duration, and onset under the age of 5 years appears to delay the development of nephropathy. Regression from microalbuminuria to normoalbuminuria is very common – up to about 10% a year, but about 20% of patients with microalbuminuria will still develop nephropathy within 7–10 years.

Progression is, not surprisingly, related to initial AER, HbA$_{1c}$, diabetes duration, blood pressure and smoking. Interestingly, progression is also

119

related to factors associated with insulin resistance – for example, low HDL, elevated triglycerides, degree of abdominal obesity, and various inflammatory markers (e.g. white blood cell count, fibrinogen).

Type 2 diabetes

Unlike type 1 diabetes, at diagnosis, up to 10% of type 2 patients already have microalbuminuria. There is a high rate of progression to overt nephropathy, about 3% a year in normoalbuminuric patients, and up to 5% in microalbuminuric patients. Ten years from diagnosis, 25% of patients have microalbuminuria, 5% macroalbuminuria, and nearly 1% have either elevated serum creatinine or are on renal replacement therapy. There is little information on spontaneous regression of microalbuminuria, but ARB treatment (see below) induces a regression rate of ~30%. As in type 1 diabetes, dyslipidaemia (low HDL, elevated apoB) and other factors associated with the insulin resistance syndrome (e.g. elevated fibrinogen) predict progression to overt nephropathy. These are important findings in relation to treatment (see below).

Other (non-diabetic) nephropathies

This remains contentious. In renal biopsy studies, up to one-third of diabetic patients with proteinuria may have non-diabetic glomerular disease, but this figure varies with the criteria used to justify biopsy. The figure in proteinuric type 2 patients selected on the basis of absent retinopathy is lower, around 10%. Many renal units screen for non-diabetic renal diseases using standard serological tests (e.g. ANF, ANCA, complement), but in routine practice renal biopsy is almost never performed these days unless these tests are strongly indicative, or there are unusual clinical features, for example:

* rapid deterioration in renal function
* suspicious urinary sediment, red cell casts
* sudden development of nephrotic syndrome
* short duration (e.g. <5 years) of otherwise uncomplicated type 1 diabetes.

Even when these features are present, in practice biopsy usually reveals typical appearances of diabetic renal disease. The clinical benefit of identifying alternative or additional renal parenchymal disease has not been established, but these are subtle matters and

120

patients with any of these atypical features should be referred for a nephrological opinion.

Erythrocyte sedimentation rate (ESR) is elevated as a result of the higher fibrinogen levels (see above) in people with proteinuria; this does not of itself signify non-diabetic renal disease.

Microscopic haematuria, sometimes heavy, is common in macro-albuminuria (prevalence estimated to be up to 70%), and is not an indicator of non-diabetic renal disease; but all patients with macro-albuminuria need a renal tract ultrasound regardless. Phase-contrast microscopy, if available, can make two important distinctions:

- red cells: diabetic nephropathy results in fragmented red cells of glomerular origin, while renal tract lesions yield intact red cells
- acanthocytes and red cell casts: if present, are more characteristic of glomerulonephritis than diabetic nephropathy.

Screening for diabetic renal disease

Type 1

Screening should start 5 years after diagnosis. All post-pubertal patients should ideally be screened annually.

Type 2

Once stable glycaemic control has been established, all patients should be screened, and thereafter annually.

Methods for screening for microalbuminuria (Table 10.1)

Arguments continue. Any timed urine specimen is troublesome for patients to collect, and compliance with producing definitive tests (timed overnight and 24-hour urine) may not be very good. The results of all methods correlate with each other reasonably closely, but this is of little help when threshold levels are critical. There is general agreement that an early morning spot urine specimen for ACR is a simple, cheap and reliable screening test, and there is a widely held view that ACR is the only measurement needed for screening, diagnosis and monitoring of response to treatment. Semiquantitative stick tests, e.g. Micral II, are now less widely used; they are relatively expensive, and at best will only be as reliable as an indicator of albumin concentration. Nevertheless,

Table 10.1 Screening methods for microalbuminuria

Screening method	Limits for microalbuminuria
24-hour urinary albumin excretion	30–299 mg/24 h
Timed (usually overnight) urinary AER	20–199 µg/min
First morning spot urine sample (20 mL) – ACR	Female, 2.5–20 mg/mmol; male, 3.5–20 mg/mmol

there is increasing interest in the reliability of spot laboratory urinary albumin concentrations.

Factors that may factitiously increase urinary albumin excretion include:

- strenuous exercise
- fever/systemic infection
- urinary tract infection (this has been questioned recently, especially if the infection is asymptomatic)
- very poor glycaemic control leading to hyperfiltration.

A positive screening test should be followed up by three timed urine samples over the next 6 weeks. If two or three of the timed urine samples are positive, then the diagnosis of microalbuminuria is confirmed. If a timed sample is used as a screening test, then only two further confirmatory tests are required. This formal procedure is particularly important in younger type 1 patients with low-level albuminuria, e.g. 30–100 mg/24 h. It should be remembered that 24-hour collections have a variability of up to 40%, so decisions on lifelong treatment must be made in a standardised way. Commonsense has a place here; heavy stick-positive proteinuria, followed by a single collection in the 'gram' range is definitive evidence of diabetic nephropathy. Albumin is stable in urine specimens at room temperature for up to 14 days, so prompt delivery to the laboratory when collected is not needed – this can help patients who need to supply several specimens over a short time span.

Macroalbuminuria

It can be argued that if a patient has consistent stick-positive protein-uria, then they are at high risk of progressing diabetic nephropathy, and that quantitation is unnecessary; such patients need vigorous cardio-vascular risk reduction and maximum angiotensin blockade, regardless of the degree of proteinuria. This is true. However, the level of albuminuria is of prognostic value: for example, in the IDNT study, the risk of developing end-stage renal failure, doubling serum creatinine, or reaching a serum creatinine of 530 µmol/L (6 mg/dL) doubled for each doubling of baseline proteinuria above 1 g/24 h. Of patients with nephrotic-range proteinuria (>4 g/day), 75–85% will reach one of these end points over a period of 4 years. Conversely, in the same study, a halving of baseline levels of proteinuria in the first year of treatment with an ARB (irbesartan) halved the risk of reaching an end point. Broadly similar results were found in the RENAAL study using losartan.

'Renoprotection' in non-microalbuminuric patients

The notion of primary prevention of diabetic renal disease with ACE inhibitor/ARB treatment is widespread. However, there were no studies to support this until 2004 (BENEDICT study). Trandolapril 2 mg daily substantially reduced the risk of developing microalbuminuria in normoalbuminuric hypertensive type 2 patients (mean BP 150/87) over 4 years. This study confirms the necessity for angiotensin blockade as first-line treatment for hypertension, with or without albuminuria, in type 2 patients, but does not permit universal use of these agents in all type 2 patients. Importantly, there are no primary prevention studies in type 1 diabetes, where non-albuminuric patients are much less likely to be hypertensive.

Management of microalbuminuria (albumin excretion rate 30–299 mg/24 h)

Microalbuminuric type 1 patients are hypertensive compared with normoalbuminuric patients. Microalbuminuric type 2 patients are likely to have other significant cardiac risk factors as well as hypertension. Management of these must be individualised.

Glycaemic control, particularly in type 1 patients, is important at this stage. HbA$_{1c}$ should be as low as possible, without hypoglycaemia, but the target should be <7.0%. CSII, where available, should be offered to motivated individuals.

The following should be monitored 6-monthly: HbA$_{1c}$, blood pressure, lipids, serum creatinine, AER.

It is important to screen carefully, especially in type 2 patients, for coronary artery disease, peripheral vascular disease, peripheral neuropathy and retinopathy. There is no need for a routine ultrasound scan of the renal tract, especially in patients with low-level microalbuminuria, but be guided by the clinical circumstances, and not dictated by the laboratory numbers – for example, ACR >~20, or 24-hour urinary AER >150–200 mg should be managed as macroalbuminuria, particularly bearing in mind the variability of the measurements; elderly patients with low-level microalbuminuria and no other microvascular complications do not need as vigorous investigation or treatment, especially with angiotensin blockade, as younger people, where overt renal disease may well develop over 10 or 20 years.

Smoking is probably an independent risk factor for microalbuminuria in both type 1 and type 2 patients; this group should be targeted actively with anti-smoking strategies.

For angiotensin blockade, see below.

Management of nephropathy

Investigations

- MSU for infection.
- Urine microscopy.
- Ultrasound scan. Normal renal length ~11 cm, weakly correlated with height and BMI; ~10 cm in South Asian and oriental subjects; kidneys are large in the poorly controlled, hyperfiltering patient, and even in advanced diabetic renal failure are not particularly small (~10 cm): cf. typically shrunken kidneys (~8 cm) of chronic glomerulonephritis, chronic pyelonephritis or interstitial nephritis. Even people with diabetes may also have adult polycystic kidney disease, though the two conditions are not particularly associated.
  - obstruction (stones, tumour, prostatic enlargement, papilla)
  - discrepancy in kidney size; if marked, i.e. >1 cm suggests renal artery stenosis (see below)
  - bladder size and residual volume (neuropathic bladder)
- Blood count, ferritin, PSA, and serum folate and B_{12} (see erythropoietin, below). Note: the normochromic EPO-associated anaemia occurs at a higher GFR than in patients with non-diabetic renal disease. Clinically this may occur when serum creatinine is only modestly elevated, e.g. 120–140 µmol/L, and under these circumstances formal estimation of glomerular filtration rate is valuable.
- Full lipid screen.

- Calcium, phosphate, alkaline phosphatase. PTH when serum creatinine >~150 µmol/L.
- Resting ECG. Any hint of ischaemia should be investigated early, though standard exercise tests may be unhelpful because of the diffuse extensive coronary artery disease that occurs in renal failure, and poor exercise tolerance. Cardiac radionuclide scanning following coronary artery calcium scoring may be valuable, but the best approach to this high-risk group of patients has not yet been clearly defined.
- Regular measurements of AER, preferably with a timed specimen (overnight or 24 hours). Increase may herald nephrotic syndrome, decrease may signify response to treatment (see above).
- GFR is an important measurement because a normal or near-normal serum creatinine may mask markedly impaired renal function. The Cockroft-Gault equation is usually used, but the MDRD equation (see Appendix) is more accurate. Manual calculation is too complicated: use a web-based calculator, e.g. http://nephron.com/mdrd/default.html or www.kidney.org/professionals/kdoqi/gfr_page.cfm

Renal artery stenosis

About 50% of cases of atherosclerotic renal artery stenosis occur in diabetes, overwhelmingly in type 2 patients. It should be suspected if there is widespread macrovascular disease and renal impairment (especially if there is associated hypertension and salt/water overload). Flash pulmonary oedema is characteristic. Asymmetrical kidneys on ultrasound should raise the index of suspicion. Duplex ultrasound and magnetic resonance arteriography are now the definitive investigations. Angiography has no place in diagnosis.

Management is controversial, and there is no evidence that outcomes are improved with surgical compared with medical intervention. However, this is a heterogeneous condition, and renal function can be stabilised, though blood pressure is unlikely to be improved, with surgical intervention. Stenting is widely used; surgical revascularisation is no longer performed.

Always consider other non-diabetic causes of hypertension, especially if the hypertension is resistant or requires multiple antihypertensive agents. Subclinical Cushing's syndrome may be present in up to 2–5% of poorly controlled overweight type 2 patients (overnight or short dexamethasone suppression test, 24-hour urinary free cortisol ×3 – random cortisol measurements are of no value), and hyperglycaemia is a frequent finding in phaeochromocytoma (24-hour urinary free catecholamines). Hypokalaemia, especially in the presence of impaired renal function or ACE inhibitor treatment should raise the suspicion of Conn's syndrome (random aldosterone:renin ratio, CT scan adrenals).

Management priorities

Specialist referral

Most guidelines suggest referral to a renal physician when serum creatinine reaches ~150 μmol/L, though some use 200 as the threshold. If GFR is used, then referral at 40–50 mL/min is proposed. Nearly all studies have confirmed that patients are usually referred far too late, with up to 30–40% of diabetic subjects fulfilling the criterion for a 'late referral', i.e. requiring renal replacement therapy within 4 months of referral. In most cases such patients arrive at the renal clinic with poorly controlled BP and lipids, and are likely to have other micro- and macrovascular complications. Remember that heavy proteinuria predicts rapid deterioration in renal function, and in these patients the referral process should start early.

Hypertension

Effective antihypertensive treatment can significantly slow the rate of fall of GFR. The target BP is <130/80 ($\cong$ABPM <120/75).

The use of agents that reduce proteinuria is mandatory; ARBs and ACE inhibitors are the only groups of drugs that reduce proteinuria more than would be expected for their degree of BP lowering. However, other groups also reduce proteinuria, e.g. thiazide and thiazide-like diuretics (for example indapamide), β-blockers, and the non-dihydropyridine calcium channel blockers (verapamil and diltiazem). Several studies have confirmed that the dihydropyridine calcium channel blockers, e.g. nifedipine, amlodipine, while effective antihypertensive agents, do not significantly reduce proteinuria. There is some evidence that statins, e.g. atorvastatin, have proteinuria-reducing effects, but in the presence of any degree of renal impairment, these patients should wherever possible already be taking appropriate statin therapy, aiming for LDL <1.7–1.8 mmol/L.

ACE inhibitor or ARB?

Wherever possible, maximum recommended doses of ACE inhibitor or ARB should be used (see Chapter 12). Maximum anti-proteinuric and BP lowering effects are seen within a month. Broadly speaking, there is more evidence for benefit of ACE inhibitors in type 1 patients, and for ARBs in type 2 patients. There are no long-term large-scale head-to-head comparisons between the two groups of agents, but small studies do not confirm the superiority of ARBs over ACE inhibitors in type 2 patients; in the largest so far reported (DETAIL study), in 250 type 2 patients with mid-range microalbuminuria (AER 46–60 µg/min, $\cong$70–90 mg/24 h) there was no difference in 5-year outcome (absolute or change in GFR) between those treated with enalapril 20 mg daily or the ARB telmisartan 80 mg daily and no difference in AER or anti-proteinuric effect. ARBs are overall better tolerated, but the incidence of hyperkalaemia, which is often a limiting factor in angiotensin blockade in diabetes, appears to be no different between the two groups of drugs (see Chapter 12).

The evidence at present would be for the scheme of treatment shown in Table 10.2.

There is recent data regarding specific agents in type 2 patients:

- In microalbuminuric patients, IRMA2 confirmed that irbesartan 300 mg daily was more effective in reducing progression to macroalbuminuria than 150 mg daily.
- In macroalbuminuric patients, irbesartan-based treatment (IDNT), 300 mg daily, or losartan (RENAAL), 100 mg daily, both reduced progression to ESRF, risk of doubling of serum creatinine, or reaching serum creatinine >530 µmol/L. Irbesartan was more effective than a regimen based on amlodipine, despite similar BP control

Table 10.2 Treatment of albuminuria using ARB or ACE inhibitor

Albuminuria (mg/24 h)	Type 1 diabetes	Type 2 diabetes
Sub-microalbuminuria (<30)	Consider ACE-I (15–30 mg/24 h)	ACE-I if hypertensive
Microalbuminuria (30–299)	ACE-I	ARB
Macroalbuminuria (>300)	ACE-I	ARB
Nephrotic syndrome	ACE-I, ARB or combination	ACE-I, ARB or combination

with the two agents. High-dose ARB treatment e.g. irbesartan 900 mg daily, appears to be safe and to have some additional anti-proteinuric effects, but these high doses are not licensed and are currently prohibitively expensive.

Many patients will require three or four agents to gain control of the hypertension. Use ambulatory blood pressure monitoring freely where available in this situation. Some of these patients will have advanced autonomic neuropathy, and recumbent (night-time) hypertension, with absence of nocturnal BP dip, is very common (this phenomenon may occur early in diabetes, even preceding the development of microalbuminuria). BP control with maximum angiotensin blockade is especially important in patients with nephrotic syndrome; about 25% of these patients can enter prolonged remission (defined as AER <600 mg/24 h).

Combination ACE inhibitor and ARB treatment
An unlicensed combination, this is nevertheless widely used. The first studies in both type 1 and 2 diabetic patients, e.g. CALM, suggested that the combination may benefit both BP and proteinuria. A subsequent study (CALM II, 2005) in microalbuminuric type 2 patients, however, found that there were no differences in BP in a group of microalbuminuric patients treated with lisinopril 20 mg plus candesartan 16 mg daily or lisinopril 40 mg daily. The best evidence for additional anti-proteinuric effects of the combination is in type 1 patients with >1 g albuminuria despite recommended doses of ACE inhibitor and diuretic, where addition of irbesartan 300 mg daily further reduced albuminuria by about 40%. Combination treatment does not appear to carry additional risks of hyperkalaemia, but the resulting near-complete blockade of the renin– angiotensin–aldosterone system is likely to compromise physiological responses to acute hypovolaemia, for example bleeding, vomiting or diarrhoea, with the risk of severe pre-renal failure; patients should be advised to stop both drugs if this occurs, and if anything more than trivial should present to A&E.

Glycaemic control

Good glycaemic control is often difficult to achieve in renal impairment as a result of:

- other diabetic complications, e.g. hypoglycaemia unawareness, gastroparesis

- decreasing insulin requirements as renal failure progresses (decreased renal insulin clearance and degradation – though it is not a reliable enough factor in clinical practice to prophylactically reduce insulin doses as renal impairment progresses, possibly in part because renal failure is itself an insulin-resistant state)
- withdrawal of metformin, which accumulates in renal impairment, resulting in a possible rebound in glycaemic control when it is withdrawn. Glitazones are probably safe up to serum creatinine 160–200 μmol/L
- sulphonylurea accumulation in renal impairment (all agents seem to be causative, even those, like glibenclamide, that are at least partly excreted in bile)
- many patients having been in long-term poor control.

Once macroalbuminuria has developed, rigorous BP control probably gives greater benefit than improving glycaemic control, and although there is evidence that patients entering renal replacement programmes with a lower HbA_{1c} have a better long-term survival, the benefits of intensive glycaemic control in chronic renal failure patients with diabetes have not been confirmed. Nevertheless, other associated microvascular complications, especially retinopathy, are likely to benefit, and there is likely to be less risk of infection, particularly important in those on dialysis.

Coronary artery disease

Subclinical coronary artery disease is extremely common (e.g. painless angina, or with atypical symptoms), and its importance cannot be overemphasised. For example, at onset of dialysis, about 30% of patients have ischaemic heart disease, and heart failure and LVH are present in about 50%. As in diabetic patients with normal renal function, the best algorithm for detection and management has not been established. Resting ECGs remain important, but many of these patients cannot undergo standard exercise tolerance tests; echocardiography, cardiac radionuclide scanning, and stress echocardiography hold out the best hope for routine detection of CAD in diabetic renal failure patients. Pre-transplantation coronary angiography is now routine, and carotid Doppler scanning should be carried out in patients with previous stroke or TIA. Associated risk factors, especially dyslipidaemia, hypertension and smoking, must be vigorously addressed.

Dyslipidaemia

Any patient with any degree of albuminuria or renal impairment must take a statin. Since this group is at the very highest risk of macrovascular complications, LDL should be as low as possible, <1.7–1.8 mmol/L. Although statins carry a higher risk of myositis with worsening renal function, in practice this is rarely a clinical problem. Ezetimibe is safe, but fibrates, especially gemfibrozil, and statin/fibrate combinations are best avoided. Lipid-lowering intervention should be early; once patients are on dialysis, the benefits even of vigorous LDL-lowering appear to be limited.

Other complications

Peripheral vascular disease

Peripheral vascular disease and neuroischaemic foot lesions are common in patients with nephropathy, and may limit vascular access for dialysis. Medial arterial calcification is usually present and widespread and may lead to spuriously high systolic blood pressure measurements on Doppler testing. The absence of foot pulses on clinical examination is the most reliable indicator of peripheral vascular disease in these patients – but the presence of peripheral oedema (stasis, venous disease, heart failure and hypoalbuminaemia) makes the evaluation of peripheral vasculature difficult. Ischaemic limbs must be assessed for suitability for angioplasty or vascular bypass.

Neuropathy

Neuropathy (somatic and autonomic) is very common, and most patients have impaired vibration perception thresholds (>25 V using the Neurothesiometer, or insensitivity to a 10 g monofilament), identifying them as having feet at risk of ulceration. Regular podiatrist supervision is important.

Retinopathy

Many patients with nephropathy have severe retinopathy; type 1 patients may have 'burnt out', inactive retinopathy, having had laser treatment in the past. Maculopathy with or without proliferative changes, with its associated risk of progressive and severe visual loss, is common in type 2 patients.

Renal bone disease

This is for specialist management, but significant bone disease can occur relatively early. If not already done, request bone screen (calcium, phosphate, alkaline phosphatase, and PTH) once serum creatinine is ~150 µmol/L. The spectrum of renal osteodystrophy is wide, from adynamic bone disease and osteomalacia, associated with low PTH levels (<16 pmol/L), to severe secondary hyperparathyroidism and classical osteitis fibrosa with high PTH levels (>32 pmol/L). This contributes to vascular calcification and increased fracture risk. The aims are to reduce the Ca × P product and to normalise PTH levels. Vitamin D analogues are used in patients with low calcium levels, and there is currently much interest in calcimimetics, e.g. cinacalcet, that significantly reduce PTH and Ca × P product in renal failure patients.

Anaemia

The normochromic anaemia of erythropoietin deficiency occurs earlier (i.e. at a higher GFR) in diabetic nephropathy than in non-diabetic renal disease. Even mild baseline anaemia correlates strongly with progression to ESRD (in the RENAAL study, Hb <13.8 predicted progression to ESRD; Hb <11.3 predicted both ESRD and death). Correcting anaemia with recombinant human EPO (rHuEPO, usually given by once- or twice-weekly subcutaneous injection) to a target Hb of ~11–12:

- improves quality of life
- reduces risk of progression to LVH in predialysis chronic renal failure patients
- decreases hospitalisation in ESRF
- may reduce incidence of cardiovascular events (RCTs are in progress).

For specialist use – blood counts must be monitored frequently to avoid polycythaemia and associated thrombotic risk – but anaemia is now an important reason for referral to the nephrology team, even in the absence of criterion GFR/serum creatinine. EPO treatment is less effective in the presence of iron deficiency, which should be corrected first. Folate and vitamin B_{12} should also be measured and corrected where necessary. Monitor BP, which can rise. Long-acting forms of EPO, e.g. darbepoietin, requiring 2-weekly or monthly administration, are now available.

Renal replacement therapy

Dialysis

In the UK, most patients receive continuous ambulatory peritoneal dialysis (CAPD) rather than haemodialysis. In the medium term (around 2 years), CAPD carries a better prognosis for survival, and preserves residual renal function better than haemodialysis. CAPD efficiency can fall after a few years, and some patients may need to be transferred to haemodialysis. Further advantages:

- Vascular access and anticoagulation are not required.
- Control of blood pressure is easier than with haemodialysis, and BP fluctuation, especially hypotension, is less marked.
- Insulin can be given with the glucose-containing dialysate, and is readily absorbed into the portal circulation – a physiological mode of delivery. Despite these advantages, this route is not usually used in practice.
- Visual impairment is not a contraindication to CAPD.
- Automated peritoneal dialysis given overnight is efficient and very convenient for patients.

Disadvantages are:

- It is less efficient than haemodialysis; symptomatic benefit is less.
- Peritonitis is common, but no more so than in non-diabetic patients treated with CAPD. Causative organisms are usually *Staphylococcus epidermidis*, *Staphylococcus aureus* and Gram-negative enteric organisms. Mild episodes can be managed at home with antibiotics, but more severe episodes require admission and parenteral antibiotics.

The decision to start dialysis is a difficult one, based on many factors, e.g. clinical factors such as presence of uraemic symptoms, and weight loss; biochemical parameters – serum creatinine 700–800, GFR <12–14 mL/min, falling albumin, hyperkalaemia.

Vascular access is usually undertaken when GFR is ~25 mL/min. The preferred radial artery is often difficult to use in diabetes, because of calcification, and an elbow fistula is often required. Everyone must be made aware of the value of the antecubital fossa vessels, so venous cannulation should be avoided at this site wherever possible in a pre-dialysis patient.

132

Renal transplantation

Selection criteria include:

- age <65 years
- absence of severe cardiovascular or cerebrovascular disease
- absence of sepsis, especially foot ulcers.

Live related kidney donations are becoming more common.

Pancreatic transplantation and islet transplantation

These procedures are very specialised, and relatively little available in the UK compared with Europe and the USA. However, both procedures, if successful, can result in quite remarkable improvements in all aspects of a patient's life. Currently they are only carried out in type 1 patients.

Pancreas-alone transplantation may carry a worse prognosis than combined pancreas/renal transplantation, and the status of this procedure is not clear at present. The results of simultaneous kidney/pancreas transplants are continuing to improve, though the surgical procedure is formidable. There is logic in pancreas after kidney transplantation.

The Edmonton protocol for islet cell transplantation, described in 2000, offers hope to a wider group of type 1 patients, particularly those with very erratic control, repeated episodes of hypoglycaemia and diabetic ketoacidosis and gastroparesis. Pilot studies are underway in the UK to demonstrate the reproducibility and applicability of this extremely complex technique. Follow-up of the Edmonton cohort has shown diasappointingly that only about 10% remained insulin-independent after 5 years, and despite the low doses of immunosuppressive drugs, side-effects were still common and troublesome.

11   NEUROPATHY

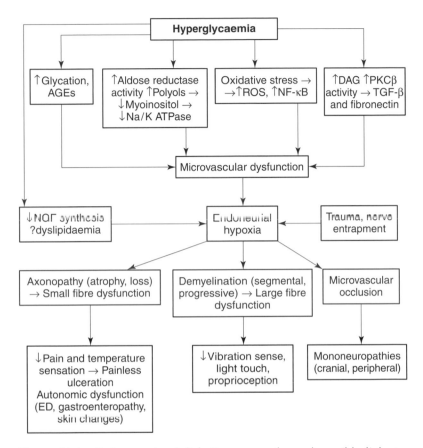

Figure 11.1 Pathogenesis of diabetic neuropathy and possible links to clinical neuropathy. AGE, advanced glycation end products; DAG diacyl-glycerol; ED, erectile dysfunction; NF-κB, nuclear factor kappa B; NGF, nerve growth factor; PKCβ, protein kinase C beta isoform; ROS, reactive oxygen species; TGF, transforming growth factor.

Diabetic neuropathy has significant consequences:

- foot ulceration
- Charcot neuroarthropathy

- pain and other sensory symptoms
- autonomic neuropathy, including erectile dysfunction.

Despite many years of research, increased understanding of the pathogenesis of diabetic neuropathy (above) has not yet translated into useful prophylactic treatment for the common polyneuropathy associated with diabetes. The development of aldose reductase inhibitors has been dogged by lack of efficacy or toxicity, nerve growth factor replacement, though logical, has not yet been shown to be of value; others have been discredited (evening primrose oil/GLA), despite experimental evidence for efficacy. There is some evidence for the efficacy of the antioxidant alpha-lipoic (thioctic) acid in alleviating the positive symptoms of diabetic neuropathy, and it is available for clinical use in some countries. Vitamins do not help unless there is documented deficiency.

Currently, the importance of detecting peripheral neuropathy is largely in terms of preventing foot ulceration, through education, good podiatric care, and footwear. On the positive side, painful diabetic neuropathy usually remits with good management, and the management of erectile dysfunction has been transformed by the introduction of the phosphodiesterase type 5 inhibitors.

Diagnosis of neuropathy

'Neuropathy' is shorthand for 'distal sensorimotor polyneuropathy'.

Symptoms

The earliest symptom is thought to be erectile dysfunction. There is insidious onset of numbness and/or paraesthesiae of toes → feet → shins. Involvement of the upper limbs is late and less pronounced – arms have shorter axons than legs. Other diagnoses should be considered if there is prominent upper limb involvement, especially if there is muscle wasting (cervical disc disease, syringomyelia).

Painless injury leads to ulceration (frequent presentation of previously undiagnosed type 2 diabetes).

Neuropathic symptoms may be intermittently present for several years before diabetic symptoms. At diagnosis, significant neuropathy (vibration perception threshold >25 V) is present in about 13% of patients (UKPDS).

Signs

There is stocking distribution sensory loss, starting with the tips of the toes, proceeding proximally, eventually, typically to mid-shin. Loss is usually to all sensory modalities:

- light touch
- pain (pinprick)
- temperature
- vibration
- proprioception.

In some patients, small fibre-mediated modalities (pain and temperature) appear to be preferentially affected, while in others the large-fibre modalities (touch, vibration and proprioception) are primarily involved.

Wasting of instrinsic muscles of the foot occurs, with 'clawing' of toes and increased exposure of pressure areas on soles. Clawing is thought to be due to motor neuropathy with wasting of the intrinsic muscles of the feet, though there may be a contribution from disruption of the plantar fascia.

Feet are often warm and well perfused with bounding pulses and distended veins (sympathetic denervation leading to increased blood flow). There is anhidrosis, demonstrated by little or no friction when the back of the examiner's hand is drawn across the sole of the foot. Hair loss is usually stated as an example of trophic changes, but it is an unreliable sign, especially in the elderly; more significant clinically is atrophy of the fibro-fatty tissue of the heel pad.

Ankle jerks are usually absent in established neuropathy. Absent knee jerks (in the absence of other neurological disease) suggests advanced neuropathy.

Quantitative and semi-quantitative measurements

Nylon monofilaments

Inability to feel the 10 g filament is associated with a high risk of progression to foot ulceration.

Vibration perception threshold

Inability to feel the vibrating head of a Neurothesiometer at >25 V when applied vertically to the pulp of the great toe has also been shown to carry a high risk of progression to neuropathic ulceration. Measurements correlate broadly with most other measurements of nerve function. Absence of vibration perception to a standard (128 Hz) tuning fork is a reliable but insensitive indicator.

Autonomic function tests

See below.

Nerve conduction studies

These are infrequently used in clinical practice, but can be useful in differentiating diabetic from other peripheral neuropathies. They are particularly valuable in the diagnosis of peripheral mononeuropathies (especially carpal tunnel syndrome) and may be of help in proximal motor neuropathy (see below). If a nerve conduction study is requested for diagnosis of carpal tunnel syndrome, it is worthwhile also asking in addition for sural sensory action potential amplitude (SAP) and common peroneal motor conduction velocity, which will give a good indication of the severity of any coexisting polyneuropathy in the lower limbs. An absent sural SAP is a good indicator of diabetic neuropathy.

All patients with a clinical diagnosis of diabetic neuropathy or previous foot ulceration should have:

- formal podiatry assessment, including a vascular assessment and assessment for orthotic footwear
- regular routine chiropody (nails and callus). Patients should be repeatedly advised against cutting their own toenails – a common precipitant of ulceration in the presence of insensitive feet
- intensive, regular education, emphasising the risks of exposing feet to painless injury:
  - always wear footwear (even, perhaps especially, when going to the toilet in the middle of the night)
  - pre-test bathwater temperature with elbow
  - check feet every day, including between the toes
  - avoid walking barefoot outside at any time, but especially on hot sand, marble floors, temple steps, etc. when on holiday – common causes of severe foot blistering and ulceration
- good glycaemic control. The incidence of peripheral and autonomic neuropathy was reduced by about 50% in the largely

primary prevention cohort of the DCCT with a 2% HbA_{1c} reduction over a mean of 6.5 years. There are no convincing studies showing improvement in neuropathy with sustained improvements in glycaemic control – other than pancreatic transplantation with resulting near-normoglycaemia which improved nerve conduction studies (but not autonomic neuropathy or clinical signs of neuropathy).

Drug treatment

No drugs have been generally licensed worldwide for use in asymptomatic diabetic polyneuropathy. Protein kinase C β inhibitors show some promise, though their primary role is likely to be in the management of retinopathy (see Chapter 9).

Foot ulceration

The ulcerated, infected and possibly gangrenous foot is a very common reason for a diabetic patient to be admitted to hospital. Most ulcers are predominantly neuropathic, but ischaemia from large-vessel lower limb disease must be carefully excluded.

Natural history

Ulceration always has three components:

- neuropathy
- tissue ischaemia – large-vessel occlusion or local trauma. Large vessels include arteries as small as digital vessels, which can become involved by septic thrombophlebitis. True microangiopathic (capillary) involvement as seen in the retina and kidney does not occur
- infection.

Additional risk factors include deformity, callus and swelling (oedema).

Neuropathy
- Loss of protective sensation (pain and thermal sensation) →
- areas of maximum pressure in the foot exposed to repeated trauma →
- callus at pressure sites, frequently the ball of the great toe or fifth toe (Plate 6) →

- ulceration: neuropathic ulcers are usually deep, clean and punched out.

The following warning features should be assessed when examining the feet:

- callus: always precedes ulceration
- blistering at pressure points, sometimes with infection
- deeply fissured dry skin, often at the heels, again a possible portal for introduction of infection
- bleeding into callus
- interdigital fungal infection
- cellulitis.

Neuropathic ulceration commonly occurs in tall, overweight males with either type 1 or type 2 diabetes. It appears to be much less common in South Asian and African-Caribbean patients (both groups have lower prevalence of abnormal vibration perception thresholds, South Asians have in addition less peripheral vascular disease and foot deformities). Ulceration of any degree always requires urgent attention by a podiatrist.

Management

Investigations

Peripheral vascular disease should be assessed. If foot pulses are present, coexisting peripheral vascular disease is not present. If pulses are absent or questionable (oedema frequently hinders clinical evaluation), then a Doppler study is helpful. If the pulse is monophasic, significant arterial disease is likely. As with ischaemia generally in diabetes, symptoms are atypical – short proximal ilio-femoral lesions that cause classical claudication are uncommon; distal multi-vessel infra-popliteal disease is characteristic.

Measure the ankle-brachial pressure index. This is the systolic pressure at the ankle (12 cm sphygmomanometer cuff just above the ankle and inflated until the posterior tibial pulse is obliterated)/(systolic pressure in the brachial artery measured in the usual way). The ratio is usually >1.0. Values <0.6–0.7 signify severe occlusive arterial disease; where there is ulceration, patients should be referred for a vascular opinion, and will require a more detailed Doppler study and arteriography.

Medial arterial calcification is widespread in diabetes, occurring in distal vessels of the foot and hand. It commonly leads to falsely elevated systolic foot pressures, and an apparently normal ankle-brachial pressure index. A normal ankle-brachial pressure index, in an ulcerated pulseless foot, indicates ischaemia that must be investigated.

Vascular reconstruction:

- Proximal lesions can be easily managed with angioplasty. Bypass surgery is now rarely needed.
- Distal disease is more difficult to manage. The techniques of subintimal angioplasty and distal reconstruction are continually improving, but outcomes are unpredictable in the individual patient.

Routine screening blood tests, including CRP/ESR, should be performed.

Take a plain foot x-ray to rule out osteomyelitis. If a sterile metal probe hits bone, then osteomyelitis is likely. The approximate site of ulceration should be indicated on X-ray request forms, so that subtle early signs are more likely to be detected.

Treatment

Podiatrists with a special interest in diabetes are the key professionals, and should always be involved in the management of patients with neuropathic ulceration. Where there is suspicion of deep infection, or spreading infection with necrosis, the surgeons should be involved early.

The mainstay of treatment is to relieve pressure from the ulcer: complete bedrest will heal most ulcers in 6–12 weeks. In practice this is rarely possible, and total contact casting, where available, allows patients to remain mobile. The technique is simple, but must be done by fully trained personnel, who understand that the methods and precautions are quite different from those used in fracture management. Poorly applied casts can themselves cause ulceration in these insensitive feet. Intensive input is required – the casts require changing at least weekly. Off-the-shelf removable casts, e.g. Aircast, are useful alternatives where individual casting is not available.

Meticulous wound care is necessary, including frequent debridement (especially of fibrinous material adherent to the base of ulcers, which delays healing and requires sharp removal with a scalpel) and appropriate dressings. Simple dressings are preferable: special dressings designed to remove exudate can be helpful, but evidence of benefit is difficult to come by. Some are designed to liquefy exudate in the ulcer cavity, and can obscure the appearance of the ulcer base.

Neuropathic ulcers should be routinely dressed daily after thorough cleaning with sterile saline. Practice varies widely, but a simple technique uses:

- an antimicrobial dressing, e.g. povidone iodine (Inadine) or nanocrystalline silver (Acticoat), covered by
- a thick protective layer of non-adherent foam, e.g. Allevyn, with a
- firmly applied conforming stretch bandage, fixed to the skin with minimal amounts of tape (these patients often have thin skin, and large amounts of tape, heavily applied, and left for long periods, can cause skin damage when removed).

Surgical debridement is usually not necessary in patients with uncomplicated foot ulceration, but where there is a lot of adherent exudate, sterile larval (maggot) treatment can give impressive results.

A member of the diabetes team, preferably armed with a digital camera (get consent to take photographs), should view ulcers in in-patients, at least every other day.

Adjunctive treatments for non-healing ulcers

Growth factors
Recombinant platelet-derived growth factor (becaplermin, 0.01% gel) may accelerate healing of chronic ulcers not responding to standard treatment.

Tissue-engineered skin
Various preparations of dermis/epidermis are available (e.g. Apligraf, Dermagraft), again with moderate effects on wound healing.

Hyperbaric oxygen
Systemic hyperbaric oxygen is widely used in the USA and Europe, but available only in a few centres in the UK. Multiple mechanisms are involved, predominantly improved oxidative killing of bacteria. Hyperbaric oxygen significantly reduces the risk of major amputation and may improve the chance of healing at 1 year. A treatment course usually lasts 20–30 days, each treatment lasting 90 minutes.

All these treatments are very expensive.

Charcot neuroarthropathy

Charcot neuroarthropathy is a destructive arthropathy with bone and joint destruction and bone fragmentation occurring in patients with profound sensory and autonomic neuropathy. It is characteristically associated with long-duration type 1 diabetes, but occurs also in type 2 diabetes. Peripheral vascular disease is usually absent, but patients frequently have other advanced microvascular complications, especially laser-treated retinopathy and nephropathy. The bones of the mid-foot are most commonly involved, but metatarsophalangeal joints are also frequently involved. A common appearance is a tarsometatarsal fracture-dislocation. When examining an acute diabetic foot, always consider a Charcot neuroarthropathy – the delay in diagnosis is often many weeks (see Plate 7).

It frequently presents as a 'hot' foot, and differentiation from acute osteomyelitis is sometimes difficult. Both processes can proceed very rapidly from a normal to a completely disorganised joint over the course of a few weeks or months. Gout should be excluded with a serum urate (but gout is unlikely to affect the mid-foot). If there is no history of ulceration, then a Charcot process is more likely than osteomyelitis. Infection usually involves metatarsals, phalanges or calcaneum, not the mid-foot.

Coexisting acute Charcot neuroarthropathy and osteomyelitis from an adjacent ulcer is uncommon, and diagnostically and therapeutically a very difficult problem. More commonly the disorganised bony anatomy of a long-standing Charcot foot leads to ulceration at a bony prominence (see Plate 7).

Chronic Charcot neuroarthropathy may be difficult to differentiate from chronic osteomyelitis, as both may show bony sclerosis, osteophytes and bony debris, but there is usually clinically evident disorganisation of the mid-foot, and although there may still be a difference in temperature between the normal and affected foot, there will be no signs of acute inflammation or infection. Up to 25% of Charcot patients will end up with a major ipsilateral amputation, and the advanced neuropathy appears itself to carry a poor prognosis – Charcot patients have a higher overall mortality rate than those with simple neuropathic ulceration. Vigorous management of all other complications is therefore needed.

143

Radiology
Plain x-ray may be characteristic. MRI scan is claimed to be the definitive radiological investigation, but the characteristic appearance that is well shown with MRI – marrow oedema – occurs in both Charcot neuroarthropathy and in osteomyelitis.

Management
Specialist input from a radiologist and orthopaedic surgeon is mandatory; management is difficult, but complete avoidance of weight bearing, preferably with total contact casting, is mandatory. Bisphosphonate treatment with a single i.v. infusion of 90 mg pamidronate reduces symptoms and markers of bone turnover/destruction, and should be given – though the long-term benefits of this treatment are not known. Higher doses are used by some, e.g. 30 mg, 60 mg and 60 mg at 2-weekly intervals, but long-term oral bisphosphonate treatment, though not formally studied, is much easier to give (e.g. alendronate [Fosamax Weekly] 70 mg), and should probably be continued indefinitely. Serum alkaline phosphatase, if elevated, will fall with bisphosphonate treatment, and is not a prognostic marker. After the acute phase, appropriate footwear is important, and surgery considered to correct deformity, especially plantar and medial bony protuberances, which predispose to ulceration. The role of more extensive surgery, involving internal fixation, is contentious, and requires highly specialised orthopaedic input.

Painful diabetic neuropathy

Painful diabetic neuropathy is common, present in 5–7.5% of a clinic population (some studies report a much higher prevalence, up to 25%). The pathophysiology is unknown, but the problem may well lie in the spinal cord. Poor glycaemic control is common, but not invariable. It is probably as common in type 1 as type 2 diabetes, but greater numbers of type 2 patients present. It is often chronic, and sometimes persists for many years.

'Insulin neuritis' occurs shortly after the start of insulin treatment. It is now uncommon, but is still occasionally seen in people with very high starting HbA_{1c} levels that are brought rapidly under control (compare insulin oedema). It resolves after a few months.

Symptoms are:

- confined to the lower legs and bilateral
- not worsened by exercise

144

- much worse at night.

  Positive symptoms are:

- stabbing/shooting/burning pains, often described in dramatic terms, e.g. red hot pokers, electric shocks
- contact hypersensitivity, especially to bedclothes
- altered sensation (allodynia) – stimuli that are not normally painful elicit pain
- heightened awareness of sensation (hyperaesthesiae)
- feeling of coldness, occasionally of warmth, in the feet
- 'tight skin'.

  Negative symptoms include:

- numbness
- deadness.

The combination of lancinating pains emanating from an apparently numb foot is characteristic and very distressing. Patients often have to hang their legs out of bed; many find relief with counterirritation, e.g. soaking their lower legs in cold water or having their legs massaged.

Management
In the presence of distal polyneuropathy, podiatric supervision and foot education are needed. The local pain team may be able to give useful advice.

Glycaemic control should be improved in type 2 patients. This usually means introducing insulin or trying to intensify insulin treatment.

Medication
Studies with many drugs have shown statistical benefit beyond the considerable placebo effect, but this is not always translated into therapeutic effect in individual patients.

Vitamins and other dietary supplements are of no value unless there is documented vitamin deficiency or alcoholism.

Simple analgesia is often surprisingly helpful, e.g. paracetamol 1 g, or co-dydramol ii at bedtime.

Other analgesics are available. Tramadol (opiate analgesic) can be started at 50 mg b.d., increasing to a maximum of 200 mg b.d. However, it should be used with caution as it has typical opiate side-effects, including dependency and tolerance. Oxycodone is similar.

Antidepressants

Antidepressants are used for their analgesic effect. All agents appear to be of value, but the tricyclics amitriptyline and imipramine are usually recommended. However:

- there is a potential for overdose in these frequently depressed patients
- anticholinergic side-effects are common
- doses need titrating (amitriptyline and imipramine 25–50 mg nocte, increasing to 100 mg)
- SSRI/SNRI agents may not be quite as effective, but carry a lower risk of side-effects and are simpler to use because of their fixed dose, e.g. fluoxetine 20 mg daily, venlafaxine 75–150 mg daily. These agents can affect the ECG (heart block, ventricular premature beats, prolonged QT interval), so the ECG should be monitored, particularly at high doses. Duloxetine, 60 mg daily, is now available in the UK.

Anticonvulsants

Standard anticonvulsants (phenytoin, carbamazepine) are still in widespread use, but they are often poorly tolerated and are probably obsolete. If used, they should be started at a low dose and increased very gradually (carbamazepine 100 mg o.d. or b.d., increasing to 600–800 mg in divided doses). The γ-aminobutyric acid (GABA) antagonist gabapentin (acting centrally at the $\alpha2_\delta$ receptor) is effective in many patients, and despite the lack of direct comparisons with other agents, the clinical impression is that it is valuable and well tolerated. The recommended starting dose is 900 mg daily, increasing to a maximum dose of about 2.4 g daily. Intuitively this seems rather rapid, especially in a chronic condition, and with a drug that carries side-effects (dizziness, somnolence, headache and diarrhoea, which occur in 10–20% of patients). It is worth trying a low dose, e.g. 300 mg daily, increasing by 300 mg increments every week until maximum relief is obtained. Recently, the combination of m/r morphine and gabapentin (approximate doses 34 mg and 2200 mg, respectively) was found to be more effective than either component alone in a short-term study. This combination, at least in the short term, should be considered in patients with very severe neuropathic pain.

Pregabalin, a gabapentin derivative, has recently been licensed for use in painful diabetic neuropathy. The effective dosage range is

300–600 mg daily, but again, it should be started at a low dose, and increased gradually. Side-effects are similar to those of gabapentin, with the addition of peripheral oedema.

Topical treatments
Opsite (semipermeable dressing), applied as a spray or a film dressing is non-pharmacological and free of side-effects. It probably acts by reducing contact discomfort and allodynia.

Topical capsaicin cream (Axsain 0.075%) is pharmacologically sound (it acts by depleting sensory nerve endings of substance P), though more troublesome to use (requires gloves and care to avoid contact with non-painful skin, mucosal surfaces and eyes). The initial substance P-depleting effect often temporarily exacerbates stinging and pain during the first days of use; the maximum effect may take several weeks.

Lignocaine patches, 5%, currently available in the USA, have recently been reported to be effective. Each patch contains 700 mg lignocaine; up to three patches, applied to the point of maximum pain, can be used for periods of 12–18 hours out of 24 hours. Isosorbide dinitrate spray (Isocard 30 mg), one spray to each leg at bedtime, may be of help.

Mononeuropathies

Peripheral mononeuropathies

Carpal tunnel syndrome (median nerve)
Carpal tunnel syndrome is very common (remember the association with primary hypothyroidism in type 1 diabetes), and may present with atypical symptoms, as it is often superimposed on diabetic polyneuropathy. The diagnosis should be considered whenever there is pain or ache in the hand or forearm, especially at night. Request median nerve conduction studies and refer for decompression. The outcome of surgical treatment appears to be equally good in diabetic and non-diabetic patients. Ulnar neuropathy is probably also associated with diabetes, but entrapment at the elbow and involvement in the forearm are difficult to separate.

The diabetic hand
In long-standing (usually type 1) diabetes, the hands are affected not only by polyneuropathy and median/ulnar mononeuropathies, but by three significant connective tissue complications:

147

- cheiroarthropathy (generalised connective tissue thickening/limited joint mobility, affecting the small joints of the hand), resulting in minor lack of mobility and inability to closely oppose the palms of the hands (prayer sign)
- Dupuytren's contracture, which is more common in diabetes
- tenosynovitis/trigger fingers.

In its advanced form, the hand is stiff, painful, immobile and weak. All but the cheiroarthropathy can be treated surgically, but an expert hand surgeon is needed to identify the most usefully treatable components.

Foot drop

Foot drop (common peroneal nerve) is uncommon.

Cranial mononeuropathies

Lateral rectus palsy (6th nerve) and painful third nerve palsy with pupillary sparing are uncommon but characteristic, again especially in long-standing type 1 patients. Spontaneous recovery occurs over several months, and they do not require further investigation unless there are atypical features, e.g. pupillary involvement.

Sensory mononeuropathy (lateral femoral cutaneous nerve – L2,3 – meralgia paraesthetica) presents with burning sensation or numbness in the anterolateral thigh, sometimes aggravated by standing or walking, with a variable associated hypoaesthetic area on examination. It is thought to be due to compression of the nerve at the inguinal ligament, and is probably more common in people with diabetes. There is no specific treatment; diagnosis itself is helpful, and there is an important distinction from proximal motor neuropathy.

Motor neuropathies

Proximal motor neuropathy

Proximal motor neuropathy (also known as diabetic amyotrophy or diabetic neuropathic cachexia) is infrequent but dramatic. It is probably a lumbo-sacral plexopathy, rather than a femoral mononeuropathy.

It nearly always occurs in men, commonly aged 50–60, often with long-standing type 2 diabetes, apparently under reasonable control on OHAs. It has a subacute onset with asymmetrical thigh weakness, with wasting of muscles and is always associated with pain – deep, aching, burning, especially at night. Profound weight loss (up to 20 kg+) and anorexia are common.

Investigate to exclude malignant disease:

- FBC, ESR/CRP, routine biochemistry
- thyroid function
- PSA
- chest, lumbar and thoracic spine x-ray.

Management

Home blood glucose measurements and HbA$_{1c}$ levels may be low, but this may be due to the profound anorexia. All patients on diet alone or diet plus OHAs should be given insulin, as it aborts weight loss and improves pain. Very low dose morning isophane or long-acting analogue should be started and metformin stopped. Once blood glucose levels have begun to increase with improved appetite, a formal basal-bolus regimen should be started and OHAs stopped.

Truncal neuropathy

This manifests as acute onset of unilateral pain in a dermatomal distribution around chest or upper abdomen, sometimes associated with weight loss, very occasionally with herniation of intercostals or abdominal muscles. It is unusual, so osteoporotic or malignant spinal collapse should be excluded in appropriate patients; shingles would be obvious. The condition usually prompts extensive intra-abdominal investigation, but cutaneous hyperaesthesia is common, and if present clinches the diagnosis. Recovery is spontaneous over several months.

Autonomic neuropathy

Asymptomatic involvement of the parasympathetic autonomic nervous system is common, but only a very small number develop debilitating gastrointestinal and bladder dysfunction, often with gustatory sweating, erectile dysfunction and postural hypotension (sympathetic involvement). In type 1 patients, this advanced syndrome, especially if there is gastrointestinal involvement, is an indication for considering pancreas/islet cell transplantation. Many of these individual symptoms are treatable. Impairment of cardiovascular reflexes is probably irreversible, once established, but fortunately of limited clinical significance, apart from a small number of cases of debilitating postural hypotension.

Diagnosis

Cardiovascular autonomic reflexes
These are the only tests routinely available for early diagnosis of autonomic neuropathy. Because there are no clear treatment options, they should be requested only when there is a clear question to be answered, e.g. establishing likely aetiology of erectile dysfunction or gastrointestinal symptoms, and in preoperative assessment of high-risk patients (see below).

Heart rate tests
These depend on the measurement of RR intervals in response to various manoeuvres (Table 11.1), and can be performed with a long single-lead ECG tracing. Computerised systems are available.

- Heart rate variation to deep breathing – sinus arrhythmia. The difference between maximum heart rate during inspiration and minimum heart rate during expiration (5 seconds each phase).
- Heart rate response to Valsalva manoeuvre. Forced expiration against a closed glottis, usually expressed as the Valsalva ratio: shortest RR interval during the manoeuvre (reflex tachycardia resulting from impeded venous return to the heart)/longest RR interval after it (compensatory bradycardia resulting from an increased cardiac output being pumped into a vasoconstricted peripheral vasculature).
- 30:15 ratio (lying:standing ratio). The longest RR interval after standing (around 30th beat)/shortest RR interval (around 15th beat).

Blood pressure tests
- Blood pressure response to standing: change in systolic BP 2 minutes after standing.
- Blood pressure response to sustained handgrip.

Management of cardiovascular autonomic neuropathy

Occasional patients have a resting tachycardia or a fixed heart rate, but these have no clinical consequences. Avoid over-frequent thyroid function testing.

Table 11.1 Values for cardiovascular autonomic tests

	Normal	Borderline	Abnormal
Heart rate tests			
Heart rate variation to deep breathing (beats/min)	≥15	11–14	≤10
Valsalva ratio	≥1.21	–	≤1.20
30:15 ratio	≥1.04	1.01–1.03	≤1.00
Blood pressure tests			
Systolic blood pressure fall 2 min after standing (mmHg)	≤10	11–29	≥30
Diastolic blood pressure rise after 5 min sustained handgrip (mmHg)	≥16	11–15	≤10

After Ewing DJ and Clarke BF. Diabetic autonomic neuropathy: a clinical viewpoint. In Dyck PJ *et al.* (eds), *Diabetic Neuropathy*, 1987, WB Saunders. Valsalva maneouvre should not be done in patients with active diabetic retinopathy.
Definite involvement: >2 abnormal tests. 'Early involvement', 1 abnormal test or 2 borderline.

Perioperative risks
Established cardiovascular autonomic neuropathy carries a higher risk of cardiopulmonary arrest in the perioperative period. The reasons are unknown – prolonged QT_c interval is a suspect – but it is wise to alert the anaesthetist to the need for close observation.

Symptomatic postural hypotension
This is uncommon, and correlates poorly with measured blood pressure fall, but can be disabling. It is usually worse in the morning. As a late complication it is often associated with diabetic nephropathy, where angiotensin blockade is required. Very careful manipulation of antihypertensive drugs is required, using low doses of long-acting agents if possible.

- Minimise use of diuretics, vasodilators and tricyclics.
- Mechanical devices designed to reduce venous pooling, e.g. graduated compression stockings, are cumbersome and poorly tolerated.
- Fludrocortisone is of value, but should be used with care, as these patients often have recumbent hypertension. It should be started at a small dose, e.g. 50 µg daily, with frequent monitoring of blood pressure and electrolytes.

151

- DDAVP (desmopressin) is anecdotally of value, but should be prescribed only by those familiar with its use in endocrinology; 0.1 mL of nasal solution or one dose of nasal spray (10 µg each) is used at bedtime. Electrolytes should be monitored frequently, e.g. every week initially, as there is a risk of hyponatraemia.
- Erythropoietin (EPO) has been used in some people with very severe postural symptoms (there is a link between autonomic neuropathy and anaemia, in the absence of diabetic nephropathy). It appears to be symptomatically beneficial, though the mechanism of action of EPO here is probably complex, and not just related to its haematological effects (increasing red cell mass does not raise BP). The nephrology team should be contacted to help out.

Other treatable aspects of autonomic neuropathy

Erectile dysfunction

The most common and probably the earliest clinical neuropathic complication, affecting 20% of men at diagnosis, increasing to 34% at 12 years (UKPDS). The relationship between peripheral neurological function and potency is weak; autonomic function tests (see above) are not usually routinely available. While there is increasing interest in the close relationship between vascular risk factors (especially smoking) and erectile dysfunction, there is little evidence that correction of risk factors improves erectile function. Fortunately, practice in this area has been revolutionised over the past 7 years by the phosphodiesterase type 5 inhibitors, which are effective and well tolerated, and most physicians, having excluded major non-diabetic and drug causes, will give these agents a trial, reserving referral for those who do not respond.

History
Distinguish between impotence (partial or complete failure of erection) and loss of libido; the latter may be psychogenic, or, more rarely, endocrine in origin. Pain (e.g. from Peyronie's disease or balanitis) may be another factor. Duration of impotence is not a useful indicator of aetiology.

Drug history
Drug history is important. The following may cause impotence:

- antihypertensives (thiazides more likely to cause impotence than β-blockers)
- psychotropics of all kinds
- alcohol, tobacco, cannabis.

Examination
- Peripheral pulses and femoral bruits.
- Knee and ankle jerks, vibration sense at feet (use Neurothesiometer for quantitative estimation, if available, though a normal vibration perception threshold does not exclude autonomic dysfunction).
- Genitalia: testicular size, penile abnormalities.
- Features of hypopituitarism.

Investigations
- Routine diabetes screening tests: HbA_{1c}, renal function, thyroid function, lipids.
- Endocrine: testosterone, LH/FSH, prolactin. Isolated low testosterone levels are common in diabetes, and should not be treated unless accompanied by elevated gonadotrophins (e.g. >10 mU/L), which suggest gonadal failure, and should be investigated separately. Remember the association between genetic haemochromatosis, hypogonadism and type 2 diabetes.

Treatment
- Any problems identified during investigation should be corrected.
- Any contributory medication should be stopped.
- Diabetic control should be improved. This was often used as an (unjustified) reason for delaying treatment, but the wide availability of the PDE5 inhibitors, which function independently of glycaemic control, means that treatment can proceed while independent attempts are made to improve diabetic control (the relief of erectile dysfunction may in some cases be a stimulus to improving self-management).

Phosphodiesterase type 5 (PDE5) inhibitors
The prototype drug, sildenafil, has been joined by two others, vardenafil, and the long-acting tadalafil. Tadalafil and vardenafil are effective within about 30 minutes, sildenafil should be taken about an hour before sexual intercourse. The only absolute contraindication to these agents is concomitant nitrate therapy (including nicorandil), carrying a

risk of severe hypotension. They should also not be taken at the same time as potent CYP3A4 inhibitors (erythromycin, ketoconazole, various antiretroviral agents, large quantities of grapefruit juice).

Side-effects common to all agents include headache, dyspepsia, nausea, visual disturbances (variable between agents), flushing, nasal congestion, back pain and myalgia. There have been intermittent reports of nonarteritic anterior ischaemic optic neuropathy (usually unilateral) occurring within hours of sildenafil use, presenting with blurred vision or visual field loss, and with variable recovery of vision. Vascular risk facors, including diabetes, are associated with this form of optic neuropathy, so the causal association is not clear.

Doses are as follows:

- sildenafil, 50, 100 mg
- tadalafil, 10, 20 mg
- vardenafil, 5, 10, 20 mg (5 mg as starting dose in those >65 years, or with severe renal or moderate hepatic impairment).

Sublingual apomorphine

Sublingual apomorphine (2, 3 mg) is less effective than the PDE5 inhibitors, but can be used in patients taking nitrates.

Other approaches

Intracavernosal injections, intra-urethral alprostadil, vacuum tumescence devices and surgical implants have their place, but are now for specialist andrological use only after documented failure of PDE5 inhibitors used properly at the maximum recommended doses.

Gastrointestinal system

Clinically, autonomic neuropathy of the gut affects only a small number of patients, but symptoms can be severe.

Gastroparesis

This is failure of the stomach to empty through vagal neuropathy. In the early stages, symptoms may only be slight fullness during or after meals. Later symptoms are episodic nausea and vomiting, leading to ketoacidosis, weight loss and malnutrition.

Gastroparesis should be considered in long-standing type 1 diabetes if glycaemic control worsens abruptly, particularly if there is unexpected hypoglycaemia (mismatch of food absorption and insulin action) or recurrent ketoacidosis precipitated by vomiting.

Management

The slowed gastric emptying should be documented, undertaken in specialist nuclear medicine departments (half-time of emptying isotope-labelled fluid and solids). Patients should have an upper GI endoscopy to exclude other, or concomitant, pathology.

Give a therapeutic trial of one of the following:

- metoclopramide 5–10 mg t.d.s. (not for patients under the age of 20)
- domperidone 10–20 mg t.d.s. before meals.

Erythromycin (acting as a motilin agonist) is effective in increasing gastric emptying, but itself can cause nausea. Dosage regimens and duration of treatment are not clear, but low-dose erythromycin suspension (e.g. 125 mg t.d.s.) has been reported to be effective and well-tolerated for several months. In-patients can be given intravenous erythromycin.

Patients with episodic vomiting should be admitted to hospital soon after onset for i.v. fluids and insulin.

Intractable cases have been successfully treated with a gastric drainage procedure (e.g. gastroenterostomy with Roux loop), but this needs careful consideration and cooperation between surgeon, radiologist and gastroenterologist. Implantable gastric pacemakers are available; referral for assessment for pancreatic or islet cell transplantation should be considered for patients with severe gastropathy and repeated admissions with deranged glycaemic control.

Large bowel involvement

Constipation is the most common abnormality, resulting from large bowel atony. Diarrhoea is episodic, lasting a few days, then remitting. Characteristically it occurs at night, when it may be associated with faecal incontinence. It is not usually associated with weight loss or malabsorption, though these may occur for unrelated reasons.

Other causes of diarrhoea should be considered, especially where there is no other evidence of autonomic neuropathy. Remember the association between coeliac disease and type 1 diabetes.

Treatment is symptomatic with codeine phosphate 30 mg or loperamide 2 mg t.d.s. or q.d.s.

155

Bacterial overgrowth may be associated. A 7–10-day course of oxytetracycline or erythromycin (each 250 mg q.d.s.) relieves symptoms in about 50% of cases. Because of the unpredictable onset of diarrhoea, patients should be supplied with a course of antibiotics to start at home as required.

Sweating abnormalities

Dry feet (efferent sympathetic cholinergic failure) predispose to skin fissuring and invasive infection. Bland moisturisers (e.g. E45 cream) may also encourage at-risk patients to examine their feet.

Gustatory sweating is rare, usually occurring in association with advanced microvascular disease, especially nephropathy. Profuse sweating of the head, neck and upper chest is provoked by eating warm food or drinking warm drinks – not necessarily hot or spicy food. When severe, it can be socially disabling.

Systemic anticholinergics or β-blockers are of little help, but glycopyrrolate (anticholinergic) used topically may be more effective. Ask the pharmacy to make up glycopyrrolate 0.5% in Cetomacrogol A (100 g). It should be applied to the affected area as required – perhaps only once every few days will be necessary.

12   HYPERTENSION

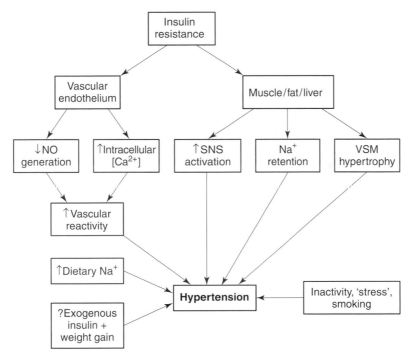

Figure 12.1   Pathogenesis of hypertension in type 2 diabetes. NO, nitric oxide; SNS, sympathetic nervous system; VSM, vascular smooth muscle.

Hypertension and type 2 diabetes are intimately linked through the phenomenon of insulin resistance/metabolic syndrome, and is extremely common – about 70% of type 2 patients with normal albumin excretion are hypertensive (BP ≥140/90), this proportion increasing to >90% in those with macroalbuminuria. Hypertension, like other conventional risk factors, approximately doubles the risk of cardiovascular disease in diabetic, compared with non-diabetic subjects. There is now general agreement:

157

- that treatment of hypertension confers more widespread benefit in type 2 diabetes than treatment of any other cardiovascular risk factors. UKPDS showed major benefits of tight control of hypertension on stroke (44% risk reduction) and heart failure (56% risk reduction) – though no significant effect on myocardial infarction – and the risk of microvascular complications was also overall reduced by 56%
- that hypertension is easier to control in the long term than glycaemia. In UKPDS there was no drift in BP throughout the trial, in contrast to the relentless climb of HbA_{1c}
- on treatment threshold levels and targets in diabetes
- on treatment priorities in terms of antihypertensive drug class. Lingering uncertainties, even in diabetes, have largely been dispelled by the results of ASCOT-BPLA (2005)
- that three or more agents are needed for adequate BP control in most hypertensive diabetic patients
- that systolic blood pressure should be the main target of treatment.

Type 1 diabetes

Patients with undetectable microalbuminuria have no greater prevalence of hypertension than age-matched non-diabetic subjects. However, 'essential' hypertension is common in both groups, and type 1 patients who gain weight as a result of intensive insulin treatment have higher blood pressure as a result of acquired characteristics of the insulin resistance syndrome (see Chapter 2). Blood pressure starts to rise at the same time, or even before, microalbuminuria occurs, and macroalbuminuric patients are nearly all hypertensive. After 15 years of type 1 diabetes, at a mean age of 32 years, 22% of patients had BP >140/90 (EURODIAB).

Retinopathy and nephropathy are both exacerbated by hypertension, and the most rigorous BP control is advised in type 1 patients with any detectable microvascular complications.

Type 2 diabetes

The same comments about micro- and macroalbuminuria in type 1 diabetes apply in type 2 diabetes, but the presence of insulin resistance markedly increases the prevalence of hypertension, especially in newly diagnosed patients.

Black patients have a particularly high prevalence of hypertension, hypertensive nephrosclerosis, and left ventricular hypertrophy – an independent predictor of coronary death. Isolated systolic hypertension (systolic BP >140, diastolic <90), associated with increased arterial stiffness, is common and serious. Atherosclerotic renal artery stenosis is more common than in non-diabetic hypertensives, but in general this is associated more with renal impairment than with hypertension (see Chapter 10).

Thresholds and targets for treatment

Type 2 diabetes

Thresholds and targets for treatment of type 2 diabetes are shown in Table 12.1. Epidemiological studies find continuously increasing cardiovascular risk above 120/70 mmHg. There is general agreement that treatment should be considered with persistent BP >140/90, with target level <130/80 (<125/75 in patients with proteinuria). These absolute levels are based on the view that type 2 diabetes is a coronary disease equivalent, and that stratification of risk is not justified in a group with an overall high prevalence of vascular disease (compare LDL levels, Chapter 13).

Table 12.1   Blood pressure treatment thresholds

Standard	BP (mmHg)	Recommending organisations
Treatment threshold	≥140/≥90	BHS-III, BHS-IV, NICE
Treatment target	<130/<80	BHS-IV, ESH/ESC, JNC VII
'Audit standard'	<140/<80	BHS-IV
GMS contract standard	<145/<85	
Proteinuria (≥1 g/24 h)	<125/75	BHS-IV

BHS, British Hypertension Society; ESC, European Society of Cardiology; ESH, European Society of Hypertension; JNC, Joint National Committee (USA).

Type 1 patients

There are no clearcut evidence-based guidelines. All patients with microalbuminuria will require treatment primarily with an angiotensin antagonist – but there is little evidence about treatment in the substantial (and growing) proportion of patients who are complication-free and

159

strictly normotensive. BHS-IV suggests treating type 1 patients >40 years old as if they had type 2 diabetes, i.e. using a threshold of >140/90.

Management

Assessment

Hypertension should be confirmed, measured sitting with an appropriate sized cuff (large adult cuff for arm circumference up to 50 cm), in relaxed surroundings without distraction, using calibrated equipment, and lowering the pressure slowly (2 mm/s). Korotkoff phase V (disappearance) is used for measurement of diastolic BP, or in those patients in which sounds can be heard to zero, phase IV (muffling). Blood pressure should be measured in both arms and the higher measurements used. At least two measurements should be taken, 1–2 minutes apart, and the initial measurement discarded. Further measurements should be taken if there is >10 mmHg difference between initial readings.

Automated measurements, especially using equipment designed for home use, are likely to be unreliable in those with bradycardia or atrial fibrillation.

Standing blood pressure should be measured in patients with known complications. Orthostatic hypotension (systolic fall $\geq$20 mmHg) is common, and may be exacerbated by drug treatment, but may not reach a maximum until 1–2 minutes after standing up. Be patient.

End-organ damage should be assessed

Microvascular
- Microalbuminuria or macroalbuminuria.
- Retinopathy.

Macrovascular
Left ventricular hypertrophy is very difficult to assess clinically. Standard ECG criteria (SV_1+RV_6 >35 mmHg; RV_5 or RV_6 >25 mmHg; or SV_1 or SV_2 >25 mmHg; ± 'strain' pattern) correlate poorly with the gold standard measurement – echocardiography – which should be requested whenever there is ECG evidence of LVH. It may be difficult to reliably distinguish between LVH and ischaemia on ECG.

Assess for peripheral vascular disease (foot pulses; carotid, renal and femoral bruits). Common and internal carotid artery intima-media

160

thickness measured on ultrasound is probably the most reliable non-invasive indicator of macrovascular disease and risk, though it is not currently widely available.

Home BP monitoring

Cheap semi-automated or fully automated machines are now widely available. Validated equipment must be used; wrist monitors are probably too unreliable, especially in the presence of atrial fibrillation, multiple ectopic beats, or bradycardia – all common in diabetes. Home BP, like ambulatory blood pressure measurements (APBM), are lower than casual clinical readings by ~10/5 mmHg. Home readings should not be used for the diagnosis of hypertension, but they are of undoubted value in monitoring response to treatment, where they may improve control. Over-frequent measuring poses similar risks as home blood glucose monitoring, especially where the results appear to have high variability.

Ambulatory blood pressure measurements (ABPM)

ABPM is useful:

- where there are variable clinic measurements
- where there is suspected 'white coat' hypertension (persistent elevated clinic measurements, but normal measurements outside the clinic setting); the 'white coat effect' is the same phenomenon in patients with treated hypertension
- where there are persistent borderline clinic values in the clearly defined 'high normal' range (130–139/85–90)
- in assessing responses to treatment, e.g. in nephropathy, in patients taking short-acting antihypertensive agents, and in assessing effectiveness of treatment overnight
- in hypertension in pregnancy.

Mean ABPM measurements correlate better with cardiovascular risk and target organ damage than casual BP readings. 'Non-dipping' (failure of nocturnal BP to fall ~10%) is associated with ↑LV mass, and ↑BP variability is also associated with increased target organ damage, independent of mean BP.

The criteria for the diagnosis of hypertension in people with diabetes using this technique, now generally agreed, are:

- 24-hour mean >130/80
- daytime mean >135/85
- night-time mean >120/75.

161

Sustained lifestyle interventions

While pharmacological treatment is needed for nearly all hypertensive diabetic patients, significant lifestyle changes will enhance the benefits of existing medication, and possibly also reduce the need for additional medication. Unfortunately, the term 'lifestyle' trivialises important and evidence-based interventions, though individual responses will vary considerably. All aspects should therefore be reinforced.

Reduce salt intake to <6 g NaCl (<2.4 g Na or <100 mmol/day). This can be monitored, with feedback to patients, if 24-hour urinary sodium or spot sodium concentrations are requested at the same time as albumin:creatinine ratios or 24-hour urinary albumin measurements. Patients should be advised to have no added salt at mealtimes; pre-packaged food and salty snacks are major culprits, as well as monosodium glutamate. The effect – reduction in urinary Na excretion by ~80 mmol/L ($\cong$4.6 g/day NaCl) – has been shown to reduce BP by an average of 5/2.7 mmHg.

Consider implementing the DASH diet. This consists of increasing consumption of fruit (but in moderation in diabetes), vegetables, legumes, beans, nuts, whole-grains and soy and decreasing saturated and total fat (further details at www.nhlbi.nih.gov/health/public/heart/hbp/dash). The effect is a reduction in systolic BP of 8–14 mmHg.

Weight loss of 10 kg may reduce systolic BP by 5–10 mmHg, though this degree of sustained weight loss is rare in practice.

The standard recommendation of 30 minutes moderate exercise most days can result in a systolic BP reduction of 4–9 mmHg.

Alcohol intake should be limited. For men, ≤21 units/week and for women, ≤14 units/week can result in a systolic BP reduction of 2–4 mmHg.

The effect of sustained implementation of this portfolio of interventions may be significant, and most studies confirm that they significantly reduce coronary risk profiles, at least in non-diabetic subjects. The benefits in diabetes are likely to be at least as great.

Pharmacological treatment (see Figure 12.2)

General points

Aspirin

Increasing numbers of studies have not clarified practice. Broadly speaking, aspirin preferentially reduces risk of myocardial infarction in

162

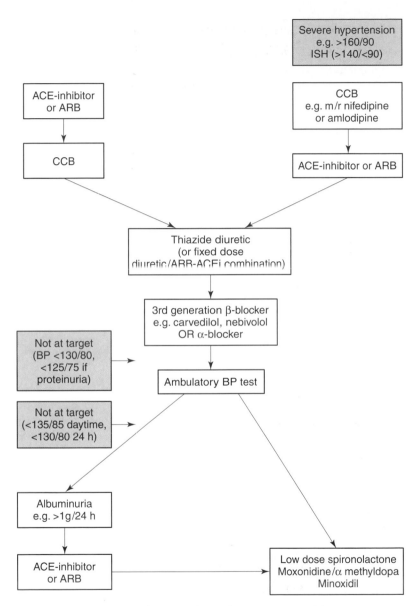

Figure 12.2 A practical approach to drug treatment of hypertension in type 2 diabetes. CCB, calcium channel blocker; ISH, isolated systolic hypertrophy.

men, and stroke risk in women. Type 2 patients >50 years old or with >10 years of known duration of diabetes who achieve BP <150/90 should take low-dose aspirin (75 mg daily), which confers ~15% CVD additional risk reduction beyond that of the antihypertensive treatment itself. It is not without risks: HOT (1998) confirmed that while the risk of fatal bleeds (including cerebral) is not increased, that of major non-fatal and minor bleeds is. The risk might not be acceptable in very low-risk patients, but few diabetic patients will fall into this group.

Type 1 diabetes

There are no clearcut guidelines. Microalbuminuric patients should have aspirin, on account of their markedly increased CVD risk, but in the absence of microalbuminuria (so therefore 'essential' hypertension) treatment should be considered in those over the age of 40.

Metabolic effects of thiazide or thiazide-like diuretics and β-blockers

Still contentious. Both classes have small effects on glycaemic control and lipids and can therefore exacerbate the metabolic syndrome. Numerically, changes in groups are small. For example, combined β-blocker and thiazide treatment increases both fasting glucose and LDL by ~0.1–0.3 mmol/L, triglycerides by ~0.2–0.5 mmol/L, and urate by 20%. HDL cholesterol falls by about 0.02–0.10 mmol/L, and serum potassium by ~10%. Newer β-blockers, e.g. carvedilol, are near-neutral metabolically. Most RCTs show significant increases in diagnosed diabetes during clinical trials, ~3–4% in people treated with thiazides or β-blockers, compared with angiotensin-blocking drugs. Drug-induced diabetes has exactly the same cardiovascular consequences as usual type 2 diabetes. However, the widespread view that they should be withheld in people with diagnosed diabetes is not rational; most patients will be taking medication for blood glucose and lipid control, and it should be simple to control for any drug-induced changes (which, although they should be carefully monitored, are likely to be imperceptible in clinical practice in individual patients). Groups of patients where they should not be used as first- or second-line agents are:

- those with the pre-existing metabolic syndrome (see Chapter 2)
- those who are borderline for a change in diabetes treatment, e.g. those about to move from diet alone to OHA or from OHA to insulin.

Once-daily medication

There is no need, with modern medication, ever to dose more often than twice daily. Compliance will suffer, and the aim should always be once-daily dosing. If short-acting medication is used, then ABPM can be useful to assess diurnal control. Regular active medication reviews are important.

Efficacy of different agents

Clinically, most agents have the same impact on blood pressure, falls being proportional to initial BP levels. Individual responsiveness will vary, but BP falls with a single agent of ~15–20/3–7 mmHg from a starting BP of ~160/90 should be expected. Recent major trials that have compared different agents have concluded that maximum recommended doses of ACE inhibitors and ARBs are slightly less effective than dihydropyridine calcium channel blockers (CCB) or thiazide/thiazide-like diuretics and that doxazosin is less effective than the thiazide-like chlortalidone. In clinical practice, such small differences are difficult to detect, and are largely irrelevant when treating to target BP levels.

First-line agents

The question of which are the preferred first-line agents in hypertension has been the subject of two major studies, ALLHAT (2002) and ASCOT-BPLA (2005). The interpretation of both, however, is complicated by the greater BP lowering effect of one regime compared with the others (chlortalidone>amlodipine>lisinopril for systolic BP, amlodipine> chlortalidone and lisinopril for diastolic BP in ALLHAT; amlodipine/ perindopril> atenolol/bendroflumethiazide in ASCOT), and the vexed question of whether the differences in achieved BP can account for the differences in cardiovascular outcomes (they probably can). ALLHAT did not contain a β-blocker arm.

In ALLHAT, ischaemic heart disease outcomes were similar in all treatment arms, but chlortalidone conferred greater benefits in heart failure and stroke outcomes in all groups (including black and diabetic patients). The results for stroke in ASCOT, however, are markedly different (calcium channel blocker [CCB]/ACE inhibitor reducing risk by 33% compared with β-blocker/thiazide), hinting at a disbenefit of at least older β-blockers such as atenolol. Likewise, in ASCOT, there were no differences between treatment groups in ischaemic heart disease outcomes. In both studies, all outcomes in diabetic patients were similar to those in non-diabetic patients.

165

VALUE (2004), comparing the ARB valsartan with amlodipine, showed that amlodipine was more effective in reducing BP, especially in the first 6 months of the study – with benefit on rates of both myocardial infarction and stroke. This confirms the view that dihydropyridine CCBs are the safest first-line agents in severely hypertensive patients, and that in the short- and medium-term at least, achieving target BP levels is by far the most important concern.

Angiotensin blockade

ACE inhibitor or ARB?

Both groups of agents are equally effective in reducing BP, and probably in reducing proteinuria and microalbuminuria, so long as maximum doses of agents are used (see Chapter 10). The cardiovascular benefits, now reported up to 6 years, of ACE inhibition beyond BP lowering in diabetic patients with known IHD (HOPE TOO) have not been replicated in studies using ARBs, or even in recent ACE-inhibitor studies (EUROPA showed benefit in non-diabetic but not diabetic patients, PEACE showed benefit in neither), suggesting that the cardiovascular benefits of any form of angiotensin blockade may not be significant in patients not at high risk (this view has been challenged). ARBs should probably be used when there is either ECG or echocardiographic evidence of LVH in view of the results of the LIFE study.

There is a widespread view that ACE inhibitors are less suitable for black patients, but trials such as AASK showed that they are effective antihypertensive agents, even where there is renal impairment, especially when combined with a low-sodium diet and a diuretic.

Both groups are metabolically neutral, and most RCTs have shown a substantial reduction in progression to diabetes, compared with β-blockers, thiazide diuretics and even CCBs. They may have an insulin-sensitising effect, and large-scale studies report an increased risk of hypoglycaemia, but this is not clinically apparent.

Concern about precipitating acute renal failure in patients with bilateral renal artery stenosis still prevents practitioners fully using these drugs (see Chapter 10). They have been associated with congenital renal abnormalities, but are probably safe up to 12 weeks of pregnancy. Nevertheless, women of child-bearing age should be specifically advised to stop taking them when pregnancy is planned and certainly as soon as it is suspected.

ACE inhibitors (Table 12.2)

Patients should be warned about cough (5–10%). There is no convincing evidence that changing from one ACE inhibitor to another is helpful. Some patients do not get classical early-onset 'cough'; a variety of upper respiratory symptoms, e.g. congestion, can occur, and the cough can be paroxysmal, delayed in onset, and slow to resolve once the ACE inhibitor has been stopped. Change to an ARB. Angioedema is uncommon, but no further ACE inhibitor (or ARB) treatment should be given if this occurs.

First-dose hypotension almost never occurs with longer-acting agents. Nevertheless, the first dose should be given at bedtime. Any loop diuretic should be stopped or reduced for 24–48 hours before the first dose of ACE inhibitor. Despite their long action, symptomatic hypotension is a common problem.

Laboratory tests

A rise in serum creatinine of up to 30% in the first 2 months of treatment is acceptable, and in fact there is evidence that such a rise preserves renal function in the long term. If serum creatinine continues to rise, then renal artery stenosis should be considered (see Chapter 10); stop the treatment, and ask for a nephrology opinion.

Table 12.2 ACE inhibitor dosages

ACE inhibitor	Number of daily doses	Starting dose (mg)	Useful therapeutic daily dose (mg)	Comments
Enalapril	1–2	5	20–40	
Lisinopril	1	5	20–40	Intermediate-acting; high doses probably best split
Perindopril	1	2	4–8	Long half-life
Quinapril	1	10	20–40	Probably best given twice daily
Ramipril	1–2	2.5	10	Long-acting. Once daily in hypertension; traditionally given twice daily in heart failure
Trandolapril	1	0.5	2-4	Long-acting

Hyperkalaemia

Hyperkalaemia (serum K^+ ≥5.6 mmol/L) is a major problem, especially in a group that already has a high prevalence of hyperkalaemia caused by type IV renal tubular acidosis (hyporeninaemic hypoaldosteronism). Angiotensin II stimulates adrenal secretion of aldosterone, and both ACE inhibitors and ARBs therefore impair urinary potassium excretion.

- Wherever possible, drugs that can exacerbate hyperkalaemia (especially NSAIDs, including COX-2 inhibitors, and β-blockers) should be discontinued. Remember calcineurin inhibitors (ciclosporin, tacrolimus), salt-substitutes, herbal preparations and over-the-counter NSAIDs.
- When calculated GFR <30 mL/min, there is a high risk of developing hyperkalaemia. In diabetes there is a significant risk of hyperkalaemia up to GFR of 90 mL/min.
- Thiazide/thiazide-like or loop diuretic should be used.
- If there is normal renal function and normal serum potassium, a single renal screen 7 days after starting angiotensin blocker treatment is sufficient.
- If starting potassium is ~≥5.0 mmol/L, or elevated creatinine or both, serum potassium should be monitored about 7 days after initiating treatment and with each dosage increase.
- Potassium levels up to 5.5 mmol/L are safe; ACE inhibitor or ARB should be discontinued if ≥5.6 mmol/L. Renal physicians are often comfortable with stable serum potassium up to 6.0 mmol/L, but at this level there is little room for manoeuvre if there is any acute deterioration in renal function.

Angiotensin receptor blockers (ARBs) (Table 12.3)

ARBs are first-line treatment in people with hypertension and left ventricular hypertrophy (LIFE study, losartan), where there was benefit in cardiovascular end points compared with an atenolol-based regimen, and there is some evidence that irbesartan may maintain sinus rhythm in patients in atrial fibrillation. All are once-daily.

Calcium channel blockers (CCBs)

CCBs are now the best 'broad spectrum' antihypertensive agents, and there is increasing clinical trial evidence that dihydropyridine CCBs

Table 12.3 ARB dosages

Angiotensin receptor blocker	Starting (maximum) dose (mg)
Candesartan	4, 8 (32)
Eprosartan	600 (800)
Irbesartan	150 (300)
Losartan	50 (100)
Olmesartan	10 (40)
Telmisartan	40 (80)
Valsartan	80 (160)

(especially nifedipine and amlodipine) can reduce the burden of coronary and carotid atheroma. Non-dihydropyridine CCBs, but not dihydropyridines, have significant antiproteinuric effects.

They are of particular importance in the following clinical settings:

- where rapid reduction of blood pressure is required (in-patient or out-patient setting) – especially where there is impaired renal function
- in isolated systolic hypertension
- as initial treatment in patients with widespread atheromatous disease before renal artery stenosis has been excluded
- where there may be suspected secondary causes of hypertension, e.g. Conn's syndrome, phaeochromocytoma (they do not interfere with renin/aldosterone or catecholamine levels or assays)
- where there is associated angina.

They have no significant adverse metabolic effects, though appear to be intermediate between thiazides and angiotensin antagonists in their tendency to precipitate diabetes in the susceptible. They are potentiated by low-dose diuretics.

High-dose dihydropyridine CCBs frequently cause symptomatic peripheral oedema and headaches. Gum hypertrophy occasionally occurs, especially with nifedipine.

Verapamil and diltiazem reduce proteinuria, though less so than ACE inhibitors or ARBs (one study showed an additional ~20% reduction in proteinuria using m/r verapamil 180 mg daily). However, m/r diltiazem does not have the same protective effect in reducing progression of micro- to macroalbuminuria as ACE inhibitors. Neither drug should be used with β-blockers. Dihydropyridine and non-dihydropyridine CCBs

Table 12.4 CCB dosages

Drug	Number of daily doses	Starting dose (mg) – once-daily unless stated otherwise	Useful daily dose range (mg)
Dihydropyridines			
m/r nifedipine*	2	20 b.d.	40–80
Long-acting nifedipine preparations, e.g. Adalat LA*	1	30	30–90
Amlodipine	1	5	5–10
Felodipine	1	5	5–10
Lacidipine	1	2	4–6
Lercanidipine	1	10	10–20
Non-dihydropyridines			
m/r diltiazem, e.g. Tildiem Retard*	2	120 b.d.	240–360
Long-acting diltiazem preparations, e.g. Tildiem LA*	1	200	200–500
m/r verapamil, e.g. Securon SR*	1–2	240	240–480

*BNF recommends that m/r or long-acting preparations of calcium-channel antagonists should be prescribed by brand name, not generically, because of variable bioavailability between brands.

can be combined, but there are no published reports of the use of this combination.

α-Blocking agents

α-Blocking agents are metabolically neutral, with perhaps minor beneficial effects on cholesterol and triglycerides. They are useful in men with symptomatic benign prostatic hypertrophy.

Modified-release doxazosin (Cardura XL), 4–8 mg daily, is the major agent of this class available in the UK. ALLHAT confirmed that it was a weaker antihypertensive agent compared with chlortalidone, and was inferior to chlortalidone in reducing cardiovascular events and episodes of heart failure. Indoramin is similar, starting at 25 mg daily, increasing in 25–50 mg increments every 2 weeks to a maximum of 200 mg daily in two to three divided doses. Prazosin should no longer be used because of tachyphylaxis.

β-Blockers

β-Blockers are unfashionable in diabetes because of adverse effects on lipid and glucose levels (see above), but were equivalent to the ACE inhibitor captopril in the small hypertension arm of the UKPDS in reducing micro- and macrovascular events, and they reduce proteinuria. Nevertheless, their poor overall side-effect profile (including erectile dysfunction), together with the outcome cautions suggested by ASCOT-BPLA, mean that at least traditional β-blockers should be regarded as fourth-line agents in diabetes, although they are not yet obsolete.

The most recently introduced ('third-generation') β-blockers are also vasodilators and are lipid and glucose/insulin neutral, and for these reasons should be considered whenever β-blockade is used in people with diabetes (apart from use in post-myocardial infarction prophylaxis, where traditional agents still have the benefit of long-term evidence – though there is a recent caution here as well).

Carvedilol, whose vasodilating properties are due to α-blockade, is widely used in heart failure. In hypertension, the starting dose is 12.5 mg daily, maximum 50 mg daily. In comparison with metoprolol (GEMINI study) it had no effect on HbA_{1c}, slightly improved insulin sensitivity and reduced progression to microalbuminuria in hypertensive type 2 patients.

Nebivolol is also lipid and glucose neutral, but vasodilates through a direct endothelial effect mediated by nitric oxide. It is given as a fixed dose of 5 mg daily.

Diuretics

Loop diuretics, with their short duration of action, are not suitable for use in hypertension, unless there is renal impairment (serum creatinine >140 μmol/L). Thiazides (bendroflumethiazide, hydrochlorothiazide) and thiazide-like diuretics (chlortalidone, indapamide) potentiate the effects of ACE inhibitors, ARBs, CCBs and β-blockers. ALLHAT confirmed that they are extremely effective antihypertensive agents, especially in black patients. 'Resistant' hypertension is often due to absence of a diuretic in the antihypertensive regimen, especially in black patients. Fixed-dose combinations, especially with ACE inhibitors and ARBs and usually containing low-dose hydrochlorothiazide, 12.5 mg, are rational and likely to increase compliance. There is a fixed-dose combination of perindopril 4 mg with very low-dose indapamide, 1.25 mg.

Use low doses, e.g. bendroflumethiazide 2.5 mg o.d., hydrochloro-thiazide 12.5 mg o.d., indapamide 2.5 mg o.d. (or m/r indapamide [Natrilix SR] 1.5 mg o.d.).

Thiazides cause elevations of serum urate and calcium, so should not be used in patients with gout or hypercalcaemia. If they are not combined with a potassium-sparing agent or ACE inhibitor/ARB, they usually cause a modest fall in serum potassium (e.g. 0.2–0.5 mmol/L), which may be clinically significant, especially in elderly patients, where there is also a risk of hyponatraemia. Erectile dysfunction is a common adverse effect.

Approach to the patient with resistant hypertension

- There should be a thorough medication review, rationalising treatment as far as possible.
- Maximise effective doses of all existing agents, especially ACE inhibitors/ARBs. Renal physicians use higher doses of ACE inhibitors than general physicians (e.g. enalapril and lisinopril 40 mg daily).
- Fixed-dose combinations should be used wherever possible, ensuring minimum dosing frequency.
- Add a thiazide or thiazide-like diuretic, especially in black patients.
- Get a dietetic review, with special attention to low-salt intake.
- Wherever possible, get a 24-hour ambulatory blood pressure test (see above). This is especially important where a patient is already taking 4 or more antihypertensive medications, before adding in uncommonly-used drugs that often have a poor side-effect profile.

If there is still poor BP control, then consider the following:

- re-consider the possibility of secondary causes of hypertension (Conn's and Cushing's syndrome, phaeochromocytoma). The likeliest cause, Conn's syndrome, is the most difficult to diagnose, especially in patients already on angiotensin blockers, diuretics and β-blockers, drugs that interfere with aldosterone and renin levels, but it is worthwhile getting a random aldosterone:renin ratio (ARR)
- combination therapy with ACE inhibitor and ARB (but see cautions in Chapter 10)

- low-dose spironolactone. Primary hyperaldosteronism may be more common than was previously thought in patients with severe 'essential' hypertension (~ 10%), but even in the absence of obvious biochemical hyperaldosteronism (most patients are normokalaemic), several studies show good BP responses to spironolactone, 12.5–25 mg daily. Serum potassium should be carefully monitored, and aldosterone antagonists not used if baseline potassium is >5.0 mmol/L. Eplerenone, a new aldosterone-receptor blocker without the anti-androgenic effects of spironolactone, is contraindicated in type 2 patients with micro-albuminuria because of high rates of hyperkalaemia (30–40% >5.5 mmol/L), and is not yet licensed for use in hypertension in the UK
- moxonidine (selective imidazoline I_1 receptor agonist). Moxonidine is probably the best tolerated of all the centrally acting agents (others include methyldopa, and clonidine – which is obsolete and should not be used). Starting dose is 200 μg daily, maximum 600 μg daily. Dry mouth and headache are the most common side-effects
- minoxidil, a very potent agent, which renal physicians use with success. However, it causes prominent fluid retention and reflex tachycardia, and must be combined with a diuretic and a β-blocker. For specialist use only.

13   LIPIDS

Dyslipidaemia in diabetes is the simplest cardiovascular risk factor to control. There are now few patients whose lipid profile cannot be optimised, or at least markedly improved, with a combination of lifestyle interventions and single or combination drug therapy. The more stringent targets for LDL cholesterol levels proposed in 2004 are also attainable – but combination therapy will be needed in many secondary prevention patients at the highest risk, and many such patients are not currently treated sufficiently actively. There is persuasive evidence that long-term low LDL levels are associated with stabilisation, or even reversal, of carotid and coronary atheroma.

Type 1 patients in good control have a lipid profile that is generally either no different from that of age-matched non-diabetic people or even slightly better (lower total and LDL cholesterol and triglycerides, higher HDL cholesterol), but there are subtle lipoprotein abnormalities (e.g. increases in small atherogenic particles) not detected on routine tests.

Type 2 patients are usually considered to have similar or slightly elevated total and LDL cholesterol levels compared with non-diabetic subjects, but recent studies (e.g. the Heart Protection Study) found lower total and LDL cholesterol; this may be because of greater awareness of dyslipidaemia among people with type 2 diabetes. Regardless, LDL levels are not significantly elevated; elevated LDL is not part of the insulin resistance syndrome (see Chapter 2). The following are characteristic of type 2 diabetes:

- increased triglycerides
- depressed HDL cholesterol
- elevated non-HDL cholesterol.

However, for a given total or LDL level, coronary risk is markedly increased in type 2 diabetes, around twofold compared with non-diabetic subjects. Whether type 2 diabetes is truly a 'coronary risk equivalent' – that is, type 2 patients with no previous macrovascular event should be considered to have as high a risk of an event as non-diabetic subjects who have already had an event – may not be quite true, but any difference between the the two groups is small. Regardless, all studies show that type 2 patients who have had a cardiovascular event

175

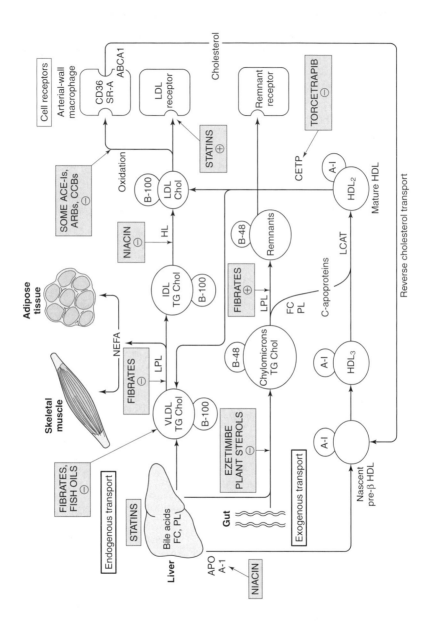

Table 13.1 Abnormalities of traditional lipid measurements in type 1 and type2 diabetes

	Total/LDL cholesterol	Triglycerides	HDL cholesterol
Well controlled			
Type 1	Normal or ↓	Normal or ↓	Normal or ↑
Type 2	Normal or ↓	↑	↓
Poorly controlled			
Type 1	↑	↑	Normal
Type 2	↑	↑ or ↑↑	↓
Nephropathy	↑ or ↑↑	↑ or ↑↑	↓

are at the highest risk, and these patients should still be the primary target of treatment.

LDL is regarded as the primary target of lipid-lowering management, with the secondary target being the abnormalities of the insulin resistance syndrome.

Non-traditional lipid measurements, which are not yet routinely available, include:

- increased apoB (reflecting the total number of atherogenic particles, which may be increased even though LDL may be normal)
- increased small, dense atherogenic LDL particles that are prone to oxidation and/or glycation
- possibly increased lipoprotein(a)
- increased non-HDL cholesterol.

Figure 13.1 Outline of lipoprotein metabolism. The function of some lipoproteins, especially LDL, is changed by glycation and oxidation, both processes occurring excessively in type 2 diabetes. The actions of major apolipoproteins and sites of action of major lipid-modifying drugs are indicated. ABCA1, adenosine triphosphate (ATP)-binding cassette transporter; ARB, angiotensin receptor blocker; CCB, calcium channel blocker; CETP, cholesteryl ester transfer protein; FC, free cholesterol; HDL, high-density lipoprotein, HL, hepatic lipase; IDL, intermediate-density lipoprotein, LCAT, lecithin:cholesteryl acyltransferase; LDL, low-density lipoprotein; LPL, lipoprotein lipase; NEFA, non-esterified fatty acids; PL, phospholipid; TG, triglyceride; VLDL, very low-density lipoprotein. Modified from Levy D and Galton D. Diabetes, Lipids, and Atherosclerosis, p.2589. In DeGroot LJ and Jameson JL (eds), *Endocrinology*, 5th edn, 2005, Elsevier Saunders.

Lipid levels in poorly controlled diabetes and effects of intensive treatment

Poorly controlled type 1 and type 2 diabetes are both insulin-deficient states, leading to markedly increased VLDL secretion and elevated serum triglycerides, and consequent increased risk of acute pancreatitis. Improvement in glycaemic control from moderately poor levels predominantly reduces triglycerides, with lesser falls in total and LDL cholesterol. HDL increases in large-scale studies, but this would not be detectable on routine testing in the individual patient. Intensified control in type 1 patients often results in weight gain, and those patients in the DCCT who had the greatest weight gain also showed an increase in total and LDL cholesterol (and systolic blood pressure), but there were no changes in triglycerides or HDL cholesterol. Nevertheless, there is concern that intensification of insulin treatment in both type 1 and type 2 diabetes may exacerbate insulin resistance, with an increased risk of atherosclerosis, in which lipid abnormalities would play a significant part, though other factors like hsCRP, which also increases with intensive therapy and weight gain in type 1 diabetes, may also be relevant.

There is little point in requesting lipid levels in severely hyperglycaemic newly diagnosed or very poorly controlled patients; leave until control has been stabilised for at least a month.

Screening for secondary causes of hyperlipidaemia

Simple screening tests will identify most secondary causes of hyperlipidaemia:

- liver function tests + γGT
- full blood count (for MCV, alcohol)
- creatinine + electrolytes
- urate
- thyroid function.

Factors modifying lipid levels in diabetes

Hypothyroidism

Untreated, overt hypothyroidism (TSH ≥10 mU/L) reduces LDL clearance. Profound hypothyroidism may result in marked hypercholesterolaemia, but in most cases of overt hypothyroidism, reduction in total cholesterol after thyroxine treatment is only modest, ~10% when total cholesterol >6.2 mmol/L. Subclinical hypothyroidism (TSH 5–10 mU/L) is not consistently associated with hypercholesterolaemia, though some studies have demonstrated improvements in lipid profile with thyroxine treatment in this group. The upper limit of normal TSH is under review – in practical terms, resistance to lipid-lowering therapy may be due to any degree of hypothyroidism. Consider thyroxine replacement therapy in patients with TSH levels consistently >5 mU/L, especially when anti-thyroid peroxidase antibodies are positive, and repeat thyroid function tests periodically in dyslipidaemic type 2 patients.

Renal impairment

Lipid abnormalities increase with progressing proteinuria, and are especially marked in nephrotic patients; the major abnormalities being raised triglycerides and lowered HDL. Surprisingly, patients with renal failure tend to have total and LDL cholesterol levels that are lower than non-renal failure patients. There is some evidence that dyslipidaemia itself may impair renal function. Renal impairment is so strongly associated with accelerated atherosclerosis that all proteinuric patients and those with any degree of renal impairment should have lipid-lowering treatment, in the first instance with a statin.

Oral hypoglycaemic agents

Sulphonylureas have no significant effects on commonly-measured lipid values.

Metformin may improve the lipid profile in patients in poor glycaemic control. There are minor beneficial effects in patients in better control, for example, small falls in total and LDL cholesterol, though no changes in HDL cholesterol or triglycerides.

Glitazones (rosiglitazone and pioglitazone) have slightly different effects on lipids.

Both cause an increase in total and LDL cholesterol level, more marked with rosiglitazone. HDL also rises with both agents, but more with pioglitazone (0.1 mmol/L, ~9% more than placebo in PROactive). Triglycerides fall with pioglitazone (0.2 mmol/L in PROactive, 0.6 mmol/L in a direct comparative study), and rise slightly with rosiglitazone.

179

Acarbose reduces triglycerides, but its beneficial effects on cardio-vascular events in the STOP-NIDDM trial in people with impaired glucose tolerance (see Chapter 2) should be noted. Presumably other, non-lipid, effects are operating.

Antihypertensive agents

For information on β-blockers and thiazide diuretics, see Chapter 12.

Coexisting primary causes of hyperlipidaemia

Familial hypercholesterolaemia

Familial hypercholesterolaemia is common, especially the heterozygous form. It should be considered in the presence of:

- premature arcus senilis (in the age group 30–40 years)
- tendon xanthomata and xanthelasmata
- family history of premature coronary artery disease (<50 years of age) in non-diabetic first-degree relatives
- predominant hypercholesterolaemia (>8.0) with normal triglycerides.

Familial combined hyperlipidaemia

This is an important but complex disorder that shares many of the features of the insulin resistance syndrome, and is the most common familial form of hyperlipidaemia in young survivors of myocardial infarction. Patients frequently therefore have elevated LDL, together with low HDL cholesterol and elevated triglycerides. Combination therapy (see below) is the appropriate treatment.

Targets for treatment

Primary target: LDL cholesterol

Table 13.2 shows the target LDL values according to various guidelines.

The concept of type 2 diabetes as a coronary disease equivalent or near-equivalent, together with the increasing number of trials that have included people both with and without vascular disease has further

Table 13.2 Target LDL values

Target LDL (mmol/L)	Guideline/ RCT, date	Clinical characteristics	Comments/ drug used
<3.0	GMS, 2003	Target for all diabetic patients	See Chapter 14
<2.6	HPS, 2003	50% with, 50% without CVD at baseline; small no. of type 1 patients	Simvastatin 40 mg daily
<2.6	NCEP ATP III*, 2001, updated 2004	Target for all diabetic patients; supports 1.7–1.8 target in patients with CVD	
~2.0	CARDS*, 2004	'Primary prevention' in type 2 patients	Atorvastatin 10 mg daily
?.0	TNT, 2005	Secondary prevention	Atorvastatin 80 mg daily
~1.7–1.8	PROVE-IT, REVERSAL, 2004	Secondary prevention; (post-ACS in PROVE-IT; stable patients requiring angiography in REVERSAL)	Atorvastatin 80 mg daily (control group pravastatin 40 mg daily)

GMS, General Medical Services (GP) contract
*See Appendix, p. 202, for websites relating to specific studies

blurred the distinction between 'primary' and 'secondary' prevention in type 2 diabetes. The best practical distinction is therefore probably between those without overt CVD, in whom the evidence would support an LDL target <2.6 mmol/L, and those who have had an event, where a value of 1.7–1.8 would be appropriate. However, epidemiologically, risk continues to fall with decreasing LDL levels, with no evidence for a 'J-shaped' curve, and in very high-risk patients, e.g. those with coronary artery bypass grafts or stents, even lower levels, if achievable without side-effects, are probably justified and RCTs will no doubt be forthcoming in due course. Using high-dose atorvastatin (80 mg daily) the REVERSAL trial, for example, showed stabilisation of coronary atheroma, and carotid intima-media thickness was reduced in the ARBITER (2002) study, using the same regimen (both studies included some patients with type 2 diabetes).

Secondary targets: triglycerides and HDL cholesterol

- Triglycerides <1.7 mmol/L.
- HDL cholesterol >1.0 (male), >1.3 (female).

At present, there is only secondary-prevention evidence for benefit of treatment of triglycerides and HDL (VA-HIT). Evidence for the benefit of 'primary' prevention with fenofibrate may come from the FIELD study (2005), though preliminary data show modest effects on lipid values, and a high proportion of on-trial concomitant treatment with statins.

Severe hypertriglyceridaemia is associated with an increased risk of acute pancreatitis, and the NCEP ATP III (2001) recommends specific treatment for values ≥5.6 mmol/L (500 mg/dL). However, pancreatitis rarely occurs until triglycerides are >10 mmol/L, at which point fibric acid drugs or niacin should be used. Lower levels can often be successfully treated with high-dose or potent statins. Alcohol and high carbohydrate diets should be managed vigorously.

Low HDL cholesterol levels

Low HDL is a powerful risk factor for CHD independent of LDL cholesterol, especially in patients with diabetes. Criteria for low HDL vary (see Chapter 2). It should be recognised as an important factor, but specific treatment is not defined, nor is a desirable level, though in practical terms, the higher the better. Niacin is the most powerful drug currently available for raising HDL levels.

Management

Diet therapy

Attempts must always be made to maximally modify lipid levels through a prudent diet. Intensive diet therapy, though punitive by most European standards, can lower LDL to nearly the same extent as statin therapy, but the necessary modifications will be difficult, especially in the long term.

General advice about dietary fats

- Saturated fat should comprise <7% of total energy intake.
- Total daily cholesterol intake should be <200 mg/day.
- *Cis*-monounsaturated fats (rapeseed, olive and peanut oils) can be

up to 20% of total energy, though carbohydrate will need restricting.

- Include dietary soluble fibre up to 10–25 g/day and 2 g/day plant stanols.
- *Trans*-saturated fatty acids (e.g. in solid vegetable oils and highly saturated fatty foods) should be restricted.

A portfolio of the following dietary components has been shown to significantly lower LDL:

- sterol-enriched margarine (1 g/1000 kcal)
- viscous fibre (~10 g/1000 kcal – oats, barley and psyllium)
- soy protein (20 g/1000 kcal – soy milk and meat analogues)
- okra and eggplant as vegetable source of fibre.

Drug treatment

Overall effects of drug classes on lipid levels (percentage change, approximate range) are shown in Table 13.3.

Table 13.3   Effects of drug classes on lipid levels (percentage changes)

Drug/nutrient class	LDL	HDL	Triglycerides
Statins	↓18–60	↑5–15	↓7–30
Fibric acids	↓0–20	↑10–20	↓20–50
Nicotinic acid (niacin)	↓5–25	↑15–35	↓20–50
Ezetimibe	↓15–20	↑5	↓10
n-3 fatty acids	↔, ↑mild	↔	↓15–35
Phytosterols/stanols	↓11–13	↔	↔

Statins

Statins inhibit 3-hydroxy-3-methylglutaryl coenzyme A (HMG-CoA) reductase, rate-limiting in hepatic cholesterol synthesis. Lower intrahepatocyte cholesterol levels upregulate LDL receptors and enhance plasma clearance of LDL. Although the major effect of the statins is to lower LDL cholesterol, the newer, longer-acting, and more powerful agents (atorvastatin and rosuvastatin) have a clinically significant effect on triglyceride and HDL levels (Table 13.4). Early secondary prevention studies (4S, CARE, LIPID) recruited few diabetic subjects, and although suggestive, the reduction in recurrent events did not reach

Table 13.4 Effect of statins on cholesterol levels

Drug	Usual starting dose (mg)	Maximum clinically effective dose (mg)	Comments: RCTs (dose used in trial)
Atorvastatin	10	80	CARDS (10 mg), ASCOT (10 mg), PROVE-IT, REVERSAL, TNT (80 mg)
Simvastatin	40	80	HPS, 4S (40 mg)
Pravastatin	40	40	LIPID, ALLHAT-LLT, CARE (40 mg)
Rosuvastatin	10	40	Start at 10 mg, increase to 20 as necessary. 40 mg under hospital advice only. Maximum 20 mg daily in South Asian patients

statistical significance. More recent studies (HPS, ALLHAT, PROSPER, and ASCOT) have recruited substantial diabetic populations, but again the results have not always been clearcut (lower initial LDL levels, heterogeneous though high-risk populations, relatively poor response of metabolic syndrome patients to statins). However, CARDS, the only 'primary prevention' study to date in diabetic subjects, has confirmed the benefit of substantial LDL reduction to ~2 mmol/L using atorvastatin 10 mg daily (major cardiovascular events reduced by 37%, all-cause mortality by 27%) in a predominantly white population with a relatively high mean baseline total cholesterol (5.4 mmol/L) and high mean HDL (1.3 mmol/L).

Dose–response relationships
The major effect of statins on LDL occurs with the first dosage step (reductions of ~35–50%); thereafter each doubling of dose reduces LDL only by a further ~6%, reductions that may not be apparent on routine clinical testing. The use of intermediate doses is therefore not logical. Atorvastatin and rosuvastatin can be taken at any time of day; the remainder should be taken at night.

Adverse effects
Liver function tests should be checked before starting and the drug used with caution if transaminases are >3× upper limit of reference range.

Periodic checks after starting treatment are usually recommended. The 80 mg dose of atorvastatin used in several recent RCTs carries a higher risk of abnormal liver function tests (but not of rhabdomyolysis), and the highest practical dose of rosuvastatin is 20 mg daily. Careful titration to achieve target LDL levels at minimum doses is therefore mandatory.

Routine monitoring of creatine kinase (CK) levels, though still recommended, is impractical, and CK should be measured only if myalgia develops – but the patient should have already stopped the drug if they have been properly informed of side-effects. If CK is >10x the upper limit of the reference range, the drug should be discontinued.

Clinical experience is that patients intolerant of one statin usually get similar symptoms with others, and if significant side-effects occur with one agent, then it is not worth trying others. Although myositis and rhabdomyolysis are the most feared complications, the most common reasons for stopping the drugs are myalgia (~5%) and gastrointestinal symptoms. The rate of all adverse effects appears to be slightly higher with rosuvastatin than other statins.

Ezetimibe

Ezetimibe is the first cholesterol absorption inhibitor, acting at a gastro-intestinal cholesterol transporter, with a mechanism of action that is quite different from that of the other lipid-lowering agents acting on the intestine, for example, resins. It acts synergistically with statins, with no evidence that it adds to the side-effect rate. Clinically, ezetimibe appears to be well tolerated, and is valuable:

- as add-on therapy to maximum-dose (or maximum tolerated) statin treatment where target LDL is not being achieved
- in patients who have a poor response to statins (ezetimibe may be particularly valuable in this group of patients, who may have a high rate of intestinal cholesterol absorption – this may include type 1 patients)
- as monotherapy when statins are not tolerated.

It is less powerful than the statins, lowering LDL by about 17% in monotherapy, and by an additional 21–22% when added to any statin. In combination with atorvastatin or simvastatin, total LDL reduction can be expected to be ~60%. Fixed-dose combinations with simvastatin (10, 20 and 40 mg) are available. It has a minor, beneficial effect on both HDL and triglycerides. The LDL effect is very likely to be

185

clinically significant, but no end-point studies have yet been completed and, unlike the statins, ezetimibe has no effects on hsCRP levels. There is a single fixed dose, 10 mg daily. It is also likely to be useful and well tolerated in other combinations, e.g. with fibrates or niacin, which are, however, currently unlicensed.

Fibrates

The fibrates (gemfibrozil, ciprofibrate, bezafibrate and fenofibrate) are PPARα agonist drugs with a broad spectrum of lipid actions, though their major clinical effects are:

- to increase HDL cholesterol and to decrease triglyceride levels
- to reduce fasting and post-prandial levels of triglyceride-rich lipoproteins
- to shift LDL from the small dense pattern to a larger, more buoyant fraction that is thought to be less atherogenic.

VA-HIT (1999) confirmed that a fibrate (gemfibrozil) was as effective in post-myocardial infarction secondary prevention as statins in patients with low-normal cholesterol (mean 4.5 mmol/L) and LDL (2.9 mmol/L), high normal triglycerides (1.8 mmol/L) but low HDL cholesterol (0.8 mmol/L). Fibrate treatment was particularly effective in diabetic and insulin-resistant patients. In practice, however, post-myocardial infarction patients will already be taking a statin, so the question is whether patients with low HDL and/or elevated triglycerides should have combination treatment with a fibrate. There are no definitive RCTs on this, but the risk of recurrent events probably warrants it in post-myocardial infarction patients.

- Gemfibrozil is obsolete; it has no effect on LDL, and probably carries a higher risk of myopathy in combination with statins, compared with the other fibrates.
- Fenofibrate reduces LDL by about 15% in patients with mixed hyperlipidaemia and reduced progression of coronary atherosclerosis in type 2 diabetes (DAIS, 2001). FIELD (2005) is investigating fenofibrate in primary prevention in type 2 diabetes.
- Bezafibrate also has secondary prevention RCT evidence (BIP, 2000).
- Fibrates can elevate serum creatinine by ~15%; this is thought to be due to increased creatinine production, and is not associated with a decrease in creatinine clearance.

- All degrees of myopathy and myositis have been reported, but they are very uncommon. As with the statins, most patients discontinue fibrates because of non-specific or gastrointestinal side-effects, rather than muscle side-effects.

Preparations include Supralip (fenofibrate) 160 mg daily and Bezalip Mono (bezafibrate) 400 mg daily.

Statin–fibrate combination therapy

Safety and efficacy have been reported in a small group of diabetic subjects with combination therapy of atorvastatin 20 mg daily and micronised fenofibrate 200 mg daily (LDL ↓46%, triglycerides ↓50%, HDL ↑22%). Combinations of fenofibrate or bezafibrate with other statins are likely to have a similar clinical profile, and although the combination is likely to be of clinical value (especially in high-risk, secondary prevention patients with a combination of elevated LDL and a typical diabetic dyslipidaemia), there is no RCT evidence to support it. There is an increased risk of myopathy, but this may have been exaggerated by experience with gemfibrozil. The combination should not be used in patients with renal impairment.

Other combinations are rational but not formally reported or licensed (e.g. fibrate + ezetimibe, fibrate + omega 3 fatty acids).

Phytosterols/phytostanols

Plant sterols, hydrogenated to stanols, can be incorporated into easily consumable fat-containing products, for example margarine, yoghurt and semi-skimmed milk. They reduce cholesterol absorption, and can lower total cholesterol by 12–14%, and LDL cholesterol by 13–16%. This is a clinically useful effect, and is in addition to all other LDL-lowering agents (including ezetimibe). The recommended intake is ~2g/day, equivalent to 1.5 tablespoonsful of margarine daily. Products available in the UK include Benecol and Flora Proactive.

n-3 polyunsaturated fatty acids

The n-3 (also known as ω-3) polyunsaturated fatty acids, are 'essential' in that they cannot be endogenously synthesised, and must be obtained from food. The major long-chain fatty acids, eicosapentanoic (EPA) and docosahexanoic (DHA) are found in greatest concentrations in the oil

187

of fatty fish. The GISSI-Prevenzione study (1999) demonstrated that daily supplementation with ~1 g DHA + EPA (Omacor) reduced sudden, presumed arrhythmic, death in post-myocardial infarction patients, without affecting conventional lipid profiles.

In higher doses (~2–3 g/day) fish oils, acting through lowering VLDL synthesis, reduce hypertriglyceridaemia by 15–20% in diabetic and non-diabetic subjects. There are no reported studies of combination therapy, though they should act synergistically with other agents, for example statins, fibrates or niacin. Fish oils are underused; there have been some concerns about worsening glycaemic control, but the effect is small and clinically not relevant.

Niacin (nicotinic acid)

Niacin (nicotinic acid), a B-complex vitamin, has a long history of use in lipid disorders, but high doses are needed with associated side-effects (flushing, itching, abnormal liver functions, elevated blood glucose levels). The recent introduction of an extended-release preparation (Niaspan) has reduced the incidence of side-effects, and the effects on blood glucose levels in short-term use are small. Its most dramatic effect is on HDL levels, which it elevates to a greater degree than any other lipid-modifying agent. It lowers triglycerides to the same degree as fibrates, and lowers LDL modestly. There is end-point secondary prevention RCT evidence in combination treatment (statin, bile-acid resins) in non-diabetic subjects after myocardial infarction, e.g. HATS, 2001.

Its therapeutic role is not well defined, but it should be considered for use in secondary prevention in combination with a statin when there is a very low HDL level ± elevated triglycerides. Gradual dose titration to a final dose of 1 g daily is achievable with a starter pack. Flushing is likely to occur, but can be reduced by:

- taking medication at bedtime
- ensuring co-therapy with aspirin
- avoiding hot food and alcohol before dosing.

Any side-effects decrease with time, but adherence to treatment may be lower than other lipid-modifying agents.

New developments

Drugs acting at novel targets are in late-stage development. The orally active cholesteryl ester transfer protein (CETP) inhibitor torcetrapib dramatically increases HDL levels, and in combination with a statin could prove an important broad-spectrum lipid-modifying combination. Acyl-CoA:cholesterol acyltransferase (ACAT) inhibitors, which have complex effects on the atherosclerotic process beyond simple lipid-modifying, are also being investigated.

14 THE MANAGEMENT OF TYPE 2 DIABETES IN PRIMARY CARE

Dr M Grenville

Background

Between 90 and 96% of patients with type 2 diabetes are cared for in the community and primarily by their GPs. The quality of that care has been, until recently, somewhat variable, but with the targets set by the government supported by the NSF published in 2001, and new treatment guidelines, the potential for improved quality of care has increased.

The Diabetes NSF has the quality of loft insulation. It is full of quality aspirations to enhance patient care – the cuddly bit – but has lots of barbs in the dated targets buried within it. The new GP contract (nGMS) has focused attention on certain measurable aspects of care for which points are awarded and these points contribute to the payments received. The National Institute for Clinical Excellence (NICE) has also produced treatment guidelines, as have many Primary Care Trusts (PCTs) to help the primary care teams treat their patients as effectively and efficiently as possible.

Diabetes UK in their input to the NSF identified their priorities as including information and education, access to integrated services, patient-centred care using care plans and annual screening to assess risk of complications.

The aim of this chapter is to demonstrate how primary care links these elements.

The NSF has 12 standards, many of which have an impact on primary care provision and which dovetail with the quality standards of the nGMS contract. The new contract has diabetes care as one of its quality standards and is worth 99 points.

Standard 1

The NHS will develop, implement and monitor strategies to reduce the risk of developing type 2 diabetes in the population as a whole and reduce the inequalities in the risk of developing type 2 diabetes.

The rise in prevalence of type 2 diabetes in the population can be reduced by tackling the epidemic of central obesity. This is particularly important in those who belong to at risk groups such as those with a predisposition due to ethnicity or family history. These risks can be reduced by supporting lifestyle changes, including diet and exercise. There is scope for this advice to be given from primary school to pension age and to people of all ethnicities. Support for the 5-a-day campaign by the primary care team is a good example, as are the proposals to ration sweet fizzy drinks in packed lunches and reduce their availability in schools.

Standard 2

The NHS will develop, implement and monitor strategies to identify people who do not know they have diabetes.

There are groups of people who are known to be at risk of developing diabetes. These include certain ethnic groups, notably South Asians and particularly those from South India, the elderly, the overweight, those who present with cardiovascular disease and women who have had gestational diabetes.

There are several key interventions that primary care can deliver.

As part of their registration check, patients are weighed and measured and their BMI automatically calculated. All patients with a BMI of 30 or more can be screened for diabetes with urinalysis or, preferably, fasting blood glucose measurement. Under nGMS the documentation of BMI attracts 3 quality points.

With the effective use of the computer in the practice, those patients with a history of gestational diabetes, previous impaired fasting glucose or impaired glucose tolerance can be regularly recalled for testing to ensure early detection of diabetes. This programme should also come with lifestyle advice to minimise cardiovascular risks. Opportunistic screening should not be undervalued and patients with heart disease, high blood pressure and abnormal lipids should be offered testing and advice.

There is a role for public health to promote public awareness of the signs and symptoms and risk factors in the media.

Standard 3

All people with diabetes will receive a service which encourages partnership in decision making, supports them in managing their diabetes and helps them to adopt and maintain a healthy lifestyle.

Where appropriate parents and carers should be fully engaged in the process. Knowledge is power.

Structured and frequent education can improve both disease management, i.e. concordance with medication and diet, and psychological well being. At every visit to the practice patient access to information should be checked and reinforced, with the offer of written or web-based material, although it is important not to overload the patient with information, particularly if there is room for conflicting opinions.

Ideally, every patient should have a personalised written care plan which includes basic information and which should be held by them. Proformas for this may be obtained from the GP/Practice nurse or the primary care organisation or Diabetes UK.

Standard 4

All adults with diabetes will receive high quality care throughout their lifetime, including support to optimise their blood glucose, blood pressure and other risk factors for developing the complications of diabetes.

Table 14.1 Reducing risk factors for complications

Risk factor	Action	Aim
Smoking	Advise to stop Refer to smoking cessation clinic	No smoking
Hyperglycaemia	Diet, exercise, appropriate drugs	HbA_{1c} <7.0%
Hypertension	Diet, exercise, drugs	BP <140/80, <125/75 if proteinuria
Dyslipidaemia	Diet, exercise, drugs	Total chol <5 mmol/L; chol/HDL ratio <5; fasting triglycerides <2.3 mmol/L
Type 2 diabetes plus another risk factor	Low-dose aspirin; and if hypertensive and BP <150/90. Consider ACE inhibitor	Reduce risk of vascular complications
Microalbuminuria	Treat with ACEi or ARB at maximum tolerated dose	Reduce risk of progression to nephropathy

This is the standard which, par excellence, impinges on all three of the areas we are dealing with. This area carries the majority of the diabetes points in the new contract as well as being the primary care focus of the NSF and uses the treatment from the guidelines.

A summary of reducing risk factors for complications is shown in Table 14.1.

Blood glucose

Improving blood glucose control reduces the risk of developing microvascular complications in both type 2 and type 1 diabetes.

Quality points (3) are awarded for the percentage of patients who have an HbA_{1c} recorded in the last 15 months. If that HbA_{1c} is ≤10%, then that award goes up to 11 points and if the control is truly good (HbA_{1c} ≤7.4%) then 16 points are awarded per patient.

Our role in primary care is regular monitoring, ensuring dietary compliance and prescribing appropriate combinations of OHAs, and in certain circumstances instituting and managing insulin treatment. The recommendation is to check the HbA_{1c} every 6 months to improve target attainment.

Blood pressure

Blood pressure is generally easier to control than blood glucose. Hypertension markedly increases the risk of developing both microvascular and macrovascular complications. Three points are available for the percentage of patients with a BP recorded in the last 15 months and, as with HbA_{1c}, the better the control the higher the reward. Optimum control defined as BP of 145/85 or lower attracts 17 points (these targets are slightly different from those recommended by the British Hypertension Society guidelines, BHS-IV, 2004; see Chapter 12).

In contrast to high blood glucose, high blood pressure is usually symptom-free and the side-effects of treatment often make the patient feel worse, so education on the necessity for keeping control of blood pressure is vital. UKPDS and other studies have shown that three medications (on average) are often required and the cocktail will generally include an ACE inhibitor or ARB.

Lipids

Reducing cholesterol reduces the risk of CHD.

As with the other tests, merely recording attracts 3 points. Control of LDL with current drugs, which are potent and relatively free of side-effects, means that this is an achievable target and good control, i.e. total cholesterol of 5 mmol/L or less, earns 6 points.

Again diet and lifestyle are vital elements for patients to enhance cholesterol control, but there is an increased impetus for giving all diabetics a statin as the target levels fall (HPS, CARDS). The full lipid profile is important; unfortunately, the current target does not yet include the insulin-resistant dyslipidaemia (i.e. elevated triglycerides with depressed HDL cholesterol), which is so prevalent in type 2 diabetes. Combination therapy is increasingly needed, especially for secondary prevention.

Smoking

Smoking cessation reduces vascular and cardiac complications

Again, 3 points are awarded for recording smoking status and 5 for cessation advice. Smoking cessation clinics have been set up throughout the UK to help smokers to quit and offer education, counselling and recommend therapy.

Podiatry

Patients with diabetes are at risk of developing vascular and neuro-pathic foot complications. The annual check should include a foot examination. Foot pulses and sensation should be checked and recorded – 3 points each. Feet should be inspected for ulcers and nail care advice given.

Annual review

The annual review is a critical component of diabetes care.

Regular recall review and re-education are vital and are likely to improve outcomes. The onus is on the practice, therefore, to ensure it has an accurate and active diabetes register (worth 6 points), in order to implement this efficiently. At annual review, patients should have urinalysis for protein; if negative, microalbumin should be measured (3 points). Measurement of the albumin:creatinine ratio on an early morning sample is the most cost-effective screening method and is available in most hospital laboratories. There are, wisely, an additional 3 points

195

Table 14.2 Annual diabetic review problems

Problem	Check	Action
History		
Symptoms of IHD	Resting ECG	Refer for ETT or cardiology opinion
Poor dietary compliance, weight gain		(Re)refer to dietician
Smoking		Refer to smoking cessation clinic
Osmotic symptoms, high glucose	Confirm HbA$_{1c}$	Step up treatment: consider insulin if maximum OHA
Examination		
Urinalysis shows blood or protein	Exclude infection	Refer diabetes clinic
BP >140/80		Management plan for hypertension
No eye review within past 12 months		Arrange eye test
Foot abnormality		Refer for podiatry
Tests		
Serum creatinine >150	Check urinalysis (for infection and	Refer to secondary care
HbA$_{1c}$ >7.5%	albumin)	Management plan
Cholesterol >5 or triglycerides >2.3 (fasting) or HDL <1		Treat dyslipidaemia, target LDL first
ACR >3.5 (male) or 2.5 (female)	Consider ↑ACR	Treat with ACEi or ARB

ETT, exercise tolerance test. Refer, ask for advice; patients do **not** always need to be seen.

to be gained for appropriate treatment of microalbuminuria with an ACE inhibitor or ARB.

Patients should also have a full set of routine screening tests at annual review, including creatinine and electrolytes to assess renal function (3 points). As well as checking fasting glucose and fasting lipids, the HbA$_{1c}$ and liver function should be checked.

Other health promotions should include offering protection against flu (another 3 points) and advice to see an optometrist or have retinal screening (5 points – see Table 14.2).

Standard 5

All children and young people will have high quality care and be assisted to optimise glucose control and physical, psychological and social development.

Standard 6

There will be a smooth transition to adult care.

Most children will have type 1 diabetes (although type 2 diabetes is becoming an increasing problem in adolescence and young adulthood) and be managed in secondary care, so most primary care interventions involve the school and other educational areas. It is imperative that teachers are taught to recognise the onset of hypoglycaemia and deal with it appropriately. Good glycaemic control is important at all stages of development, especially during adolescence. Children and their families should be educated to this end and there are now interactive and web-based educational programmes available.

Transfer of care to the adult sector should be carefully planned, though this can be a difficult transition, and primary care can play an important active role here. Dedicated young adult clinics in secondary care can also be useful.

Standard 7

There are standard protocols for the management of diabetic emergencies.

There should be in all accident and emergency departments a protocol to manage diabetic emergencies.

The early recognition of hyperglycaemic emergencies is important as many newly diagnosed type 1 diabetics present in primary care. Urinalysis for ketones and urgent referral to A&E or the hospital-based diabetes team can be life saving.

Within the primary care setting, the patient-held care plan should contain guidance on the management of changes in blood glucose. 'Sick day rules', for example, can reduce the risk and severity of ketoacidosis. Recognition of frequent hypoglycaemia (in both type 1 and type 2 patients) is important. Insulin-managed patients will require a dose reduction and rapid referral to the secondary care diabetes nurse specialist.

Standard 8

Diabetic patients on admission to hospital will receive appropriate care and supervision whatever the reason for hospitalisation.

Standard 9

Women with diabetes who become pregnant will get appropriate support and care.

These are also hospital-based standards but ensuring full information is given in any referrals can help improve the quality of perioperative care that can be given; GP teams can also support the very important link between ward teams and hospital diabetes teams.

Sound contraceptive advice is important for all women with diabetes and every effort should be made to avoid an unplanned pregnancy. Pre-pregnancy counselling and rapid referral to the appropriate secondary care team is critical and will improve pregnancy outcomes. It is also important to inform the practices when patients develop gestational diabetes so ongoing, structured follow-up and screening can be arranged. These women are at very high risk of developing permanent type 2 diabetes, and are rarely followed closely in secondary care once they have delivered.

Standard 10

All young people will receive regular surveillance for complications.

Standard 11

People who develop complications will receive timely, appropriate and effective treatment to reduce disability and premature death.

Most microvascular complications could and should be picked up at review sessions, hence the importance of regular podiatrist and optometrist review.

The NSF-led introduction of comprehensive digital retinal photographic surveillance should result in lower rates of visual loss from retinopathy.

Good foot care and referral of patients with clinical neuropathy to the podiatry service can have an impact on the development of neuropathic foot ulcers, a costly complication.

Annual renal screening will allow the rapid referral of patients with a rising serum creatinine (>150 μmol/L) and increasing proteinuria to the local diabetes/renal team, in order to avoid late referrals requiring hazardous and rapid institution of renal replacement therapy. Renal complications can be retarded by treatment of microalbuminuria with ACE inhibitor or ARBs.

Tight BP and lipid control can reduce the risks of macrovascular complications and coronary disease. Patients who suffer a myocardial infarction will require vigorous risk reduction, and although most of the drugs will be initiated in secondary care, the role of the primary care team in reinforcing treatment adherence and lifestyle changes is crucial.

Standard 12

All people will receive integrated health and social care.

Within primary care we have the tools to look after type 2 diabetes to a high standard, with demonstrable reductions in end-stage complications, especially coronary artery disease. By running a system that ensures regular call and recall of diabetic patients with a method of chasing non-attenders (who are likely to have the highest risks of micro- and macrovascular disease) and by using education as a motivator, we can bring many (if not most) of our patients into a state of good health. If we undertake full annual checks with appropriate 6-monthly blood and urine tests and, following guidelines, treat appropriately without being afraid of multiple therapy, then we can keep stable patients in primary care. This of course leaves scope for referring complex patients with multiple complications for early hospital evaluation.

APPENDIX: SOURCES AND WEBSITES

National diabetes organisations

- Diabetes UK: diabetes.org.uk
- American Diabetes Association: diabetes.org
- Diabetes Australia: diabetesaustralia.com.au
- Diabetes New Zealand: diabetes.org.nz
- Canadian Diabetes Association: diabetes.ca
- Association of British Clinical Diabetologists (ABCD): diabetologists.org.uk

Other national organisations

- British Hypertension Society: bhsoc.org
- British Heart Foundation: bhf.org.uk
  Statistics website: heartstats.org
- Joint British Societies Cardiac Risk Assessor (MS Excel): bnf.org/bnf/extra/50/openat/450024.htm (also creatinine clearance calculator)
- Medline, through National Institutes of Health: nlm.nih.gov
- National Service Framework (NSF) for diabetes: dh.gov.uk/PolicyAndGuidance/HealthAndSocialCareTopics/Diabetes/fs/en

Guidelines

Scottish Intercollegiate Guidelines Network (SIGN): sign.ac.uk

Many of the national diabetes organisation websites contain guidelines. In the UK, comprehensive guidelines are published by SIGN; their diabetes guidelines (No 55: Management of Diabetes) were last revised November 2001 (sign.ac.uk/guidelines/fulltext/55/index.html).

National Institute for Health and Clinical Excellence (NICE): nice.org.uk

NICE publishes both Technology Appraisals relating to individual drugs, drug groups, devices or procedures, and Clinical Guidelines.

Technology Appraisals related to diabetes:

- Insulin pump therapy (2003)
- Glitazones (2003, review 2006)
- Long-acting insulin analogues (2002, review 2005)
- Diabetes (types 1 and 2) – inhaled insulin (2006)
- Patient education models (2003, review 2006)
- Diabetes in pregnancy (due 2008)
- Cardiovascular risk assessment (lipids, due 2007)

Several major (book-length) evidence-based Clinical Guidelines were published in 2004:

- Type 1 diabetes: diagnosis and management of type 1 diabetes in adults
- Type 1 diabetes: diagnosis and management of type 1 diabetes in children and young adults
- Type 2 diabetes: footcare (2004)
- Inherited guidelines on type 2 diabetes (blood glucose, blood pressure, lipids, renal disease, retinopathy)
- Full type 2 diabetes guidelines (in development from 2006)

Websites relating to specific clinical studies

Some of these sites include PowerPoint presentations of the trial designs and outcomes, and some can be downloaded for personal use.

- ALLHAT: http://allhat.sph.uth.tmc.edu
- CARDS: cardstrial.org
- DCCT/EDIC: diabetes.niddk.nih.gov/ (homepage; DCCT/EDIC slides not available)
- PROactive: proactive-results.com
- UKPDS: dtu.ox.ac.uk/ukpds/
- Clinical Trial Results: clinicaltrialresults.org (current cardiology clinical trial results presented at major international meetings; all presentations downloadable; a valuable resource)

- NCEP ATP III (National Cholesterol Education Program Adult Treatment Panel III 2001) – guidelines on lipid management (USA): nhlbi.nih.gov/guidelines/cholesterol/
- inCirculation.net (cardiovascular website with extensive links, sponsored by AstraZeneca)

Specialist diabetes/endocrinology websites

- Medscape.com
- CMEonDiabetes.com (associated website on matters relating to CRP – CRPhealth.com)
- lipidsonline.org (Baylor College of Medicine)
- National Diabetes Education Initiative: ndei.org

Registration is required for some of these sites, but there are outstanding academic and practical updates, with on-line lectures from major meetings, especially the American Diabetes Association Scientific Sessions. CRPhealth.com has downloadable journal articles and PowerPoint slide presentations.

UK diabetes centre websites

- West Sussex Diabetes Service: diabetesuffolk.com
- Bournemouth Diabetes & Endocrine Centre: b-dec.com

Insulin pump users organisation

- insulin-pumpers.org.uk

Online GFR calculation

- kidney.org.professionals/kdoqi/gfr_page.cfm
- http://nephron.com/mdrd/default.html

203

INDEX

Note: page numbers in *italics* refer to figures and tables

208

PRACTICAL DIABETES